The Calculation of Genetic Risks

Peter J. Bridge —————————————

The Calculation
of Genetic Risks

WORKED EXAMPLES IN
DNA DIAGNOSTICS

THE JOHNS HOPKINS UNIVERSITY PRESS

BALTIMORE AND LONDON

The Johns Hopkins University Press
2715 North Charles Street
Baltimore, Maryland 21218-4319
The Johns Hopkins Press Ltd., London

Library of Congress Cataloging-in-Publication Data
will be found at the end of this book.

A catalog record for this book is available
from the British Library.

DEDICATION

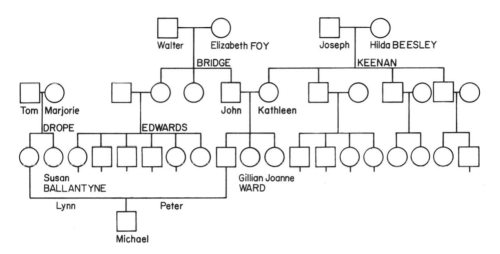

Contents

Acknowledgments

I wish to acknowledge all those who have helped directly or indirectly over the years in the work that led to the preparation of this text. In particular, Helmut Bertrand and Rod Kelln, who taught me genetics and challenged the development of critical thinking during my graduate studies at the University of Regina; David Lillicrap, co-director of the DNA Diagnostic Laboratory at Kingston General Hospital, and Patrick MacLeod, clinical geneticist; technologists Colleen Clarke, Rena D'Souza, Jane Lovsted, Larry Weiler, and Sharon Windsor; graduate students Gail Graham and Paul Wilkins; postdoctoral fellow Nancy Carson; summer students Karen Kong and Peter Schuringa; artist Sue Hoyle; and secretaries Lorrie Casford and Hermina Wensing. Finally, I must acknowledge the patient guidance and encouragement of Wendy Harris, medical editor, Johns Hopkins University Press. Without the guidance, dedicated professionalism, and friendship of these people, the picture below would not be just a joke.

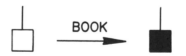

I thank Drs. Tony Round, Stephen Wood, Nancy Carson, and anonymous reviewers for their valuable comments on various drafts of this book. Any errors that remain, of course, are my responsibility. I must commend the vision of several Canadian provincial governments and their genetic advisory committees in seeing the need for molecular diagnostic laboratories several years ago and fully underwriting the cost of their development and operation for the benefit of all.

Statement on Discrimination

There is a valid need for educators in almost all settings to strive to be, and to be perceived to be, nondiscriminatory in matters pertaining to age, race, religion, gender, sexual orientation, political affiliation, and so forth. To this list we should add genotype. Medical genetics studies people's genotypes and the effects that such genotypes have upon their lives. The bulk of this book is devoted to methods that can be used to determine or predict people's genotypes. The information gained by such processes must be used only for the benefit of that person and only with his or her explicit informed consent, usually in the attempt to answer a private and personal question.

The information derived from DNA studies has far-reaching consequences: it is different from almost all other types of medical information in that (a) it has predictive value rather than being just a historical record of a person's health to date and (b) the knowledge of one person's genotype automatically gives away information about relatives with or without their consent or active participation. For these reasons, genotypic data must be guarded with the utmost confidentiality, used prudently, and kept out of medical records until a fail-safe mechanism has been developed and fully implemented that guarantees that predictive information on an individual and the inevitably associated family group cannot be used against them. At this time, the vast majority of physicians and other professionals do not understand fully the implications that the knowledge of one person's genotype can carry for others. As an extreme example, can we afford to have a bright defense lawyer plead that his 35-year-old male client was biologically compelled to rob the bank because he is a transmitting male for fragile X syndrome and (in addition to losing the case) then find out later that his client's five daughters are unable to obtain medical insurance policies? Genetic information is a bit like nuclear warfare: we are all in it together. Ways must be developed that will allow us to provide freely the information that will help the person in our office today and yet prevent the unintentional but concomitant divulgence of unauthorized information pertaining to others. Given the current laws of many countries regarding access to medical information, this is a very urgent matter.

The philosophy of nondiscrimination, while laudable in general, can also be overzealously applied. As an example, in 1990, some well-meaning official at a Ministry of Health that I will not name read through the final draft of a pamphlet on amniocentesis immediately before thousands of copies were to be printed, deleted late maternal age as an indication for amniocentesis because it discriminates on the basis of age and on the basis of gender, and sent the modified text to the printer without informing the panel of medical geneticists who wrote the pamphlet of the change. Let us be thankful that the same well-meaning but misguided official did not proofread any information packages on mammography or prostate surgery. There are obviously many situations where it is both appropriate and necessary to be specific: technical specificity should not be equated with discrimination.

This book discusses, on probably half of its pages, people of different genders in gender-specific ways and, on a few occasions, people of different races in race-specific ways. Nothing negative or derogatory is implied or intended, just an honest discussion of X and Y chromosomes and our genetic heritage.

Introduction

I went into a hamburger restaurant a little while ago and ordered a sumptuous meal for two, totaling $11.34. I gave the young man who took the order $21.34 (a $20 bill and $1.34 in coins), since I wanted to lighten the burden on my pockets rather than receive even more coins. As is a common antitheft policy in such institutions, he hid the $20 under the tray containing the coins, and since he knew that the $20 was more than enough, he could not figure out why I had given him extra money in the form of all those coins. I don't know what grade he was in, but he obviously could not add change, and next he took the coins to the shift supervisor, asked her how much I had given him, and obtained the correct answer of $1.34. Satisfied, and forgetting my $20 bill, he typed $1.34 as the amount tendered into the computer in front of him, and never batted an eyelid when it told him that I still owed $10.00. His confident demand for another $10 and my howl of protest rapidly brought the shift supervisor to the scene, who, although she had added up $1.34 very efficiently, left something to be desired in comprehending the fate of the $20 bill.

Has anything like this ever happened to you? The electronic part of the team performed faultlessly but was operated by someone who lacked the basic skills to tell that it had been asked the wrong question.

Modern jet aircraft are wonders of technical wizardry. They are flown most of the time by complex autopilot programs. It is very reassuring, however, for us passengers to know that if, for whatever reason, something goes wrong with this electronic marvel, we can count on the captain to get us there safely. This assumes, of course, that the captain can actually fly the aircraft without using the autopilot, should this become necessary. Wind shear, cabin depressurization, and tires bursting on takeoff perhaps have their equivalents lurking in the molecular diagnostics laboratory. As exotic examples, gene conversion and uniparental disomy are not programmed into the current generation of risk-calculating programs, nor are more mundane problems such as mosaicism or maternal cell contamination. If the operator does not know the characteristics of such nonroutine events, they will escape consideration, let alone detection.

Particularly disturbing, however, is the fact that the literature is replete with senseless data that escape challenge or further scrutiny because of the assumption that computers do not make mistakes. Although this assumption may well be true if they are correctly programed and supplied with error-free input, unfortunately it seems that in a number of cases the operator is unable to tell the difference. The numerical data presented in any paper that mentions the use of one of the well-known computer programs as the means by which the linkage calculations were performed seem to escape the careful scrutiny that expert reviewers and editors apply so thoroughly to the text and artwork. To pick but one example out of very many, how else can we explain statements such as "One recombination event was observed . . . in 36 informative meioses . . . giving a peak lod score of 5.86 at a corresponding recombination fraction of .00" (*American Journal of Human Genetics,* 1989, in boldface type in the Abstract) and "one recombination event was observed among 36 informative meioses, and a peak lod score (Zmax) of 5.86 was calculated (peak recombination fraction [θmax] = 0.00)" (same paper, in the Results section). The fact that the error is repeated probably indicates that it is not a typographical error on the part of the journal. I think that we can reasonably grant that the editors and expert reviewers for a prestigious journal know that θmax cannot be 0.00 if recombinants were detected, which leads to the conclusion that the data were accepted without being read.

The basic aim of this book is to impart to the reader the fundamentals of how we start with laboratory results and end up with numbers representing genetic risks. The aim will never be to be mathematically correct to many decimal places nor to avoid the use of the complex computer programs that can generate risks correct to about the tenth decimal place when programed correctly and used appropriately. If, however, it imparts enough theory and gives enough practice through the use of worked examples so that readers can critically assess either a published manuscript or the risk assigned to a family member and say, "Yes, I agree with this," or "No, this is clearly incorrect," then I believe that they will be better suited for the responsibility of providing a good-quality genetic service that the public entrusts to them.

This book is not filled with abstract equations; they mean little to me and I suspect also to the majority of people in the field of medical genetics. Instead, it concentrates upon worked examples using numbers instead of symbols. What it lacks in mathematical grace, I hope it makes up for in intelligibility.

The book starts with a detailed discussion of Bayesian calculations and pedigree risks, for two reasons: (a) to set the general framework for approaches to risk calculations and (b) in later chapters when we use DNA markers, to show the contrast created when we know which of the two copies of a gene was actually or probably inherited (predictive versus descriptive). Although not every scenario can be covered, I hope that I provide examples of a sufficiently diverse spectrum of permutations of pedigree and RFLP data with new mutations, biochemical test results, incomplete penetrance, and so forth, for readers to be able to create constructive approaches to whatever specific situations confront them.

Finally, I have deliberately chosen to write a book about the process rather than the specifics. Rather than write about specific diseases and studies with specific markers, I have tried wherever possible to write about generic examples. I have deliberately tried to steer away from examples that appear to give specific advice about which markers would be suitable for a specific disease, because such choices will obviously change over time. Similarly, in the sample calculations I have sometimes had to pick a number to use, such as assuming that one in three carriers of Duchenne muscular dystrophy has "normal" levels of creatine kinase in their blood and that one in twenty noncarriers has "abnormal" levels; the actual numbers that you should use clearly must be the false-negative and false-positive rates quoted by the laboratory that did your analysis.

The Calculation of Genetic Risks

1

General Introduction to

the Estimation of Genetic Risks

Genetic risks for single-gene (Mendelian) disorders are, on the whole, relatively straightforward to calculate. For instance, to start at the easy end of the spectrum, a prospective parent with an autosomal dominant condition has a 50% risk of passing the mutant allele to each child. Similarly, the recurrence risk for the next pregnancy of a couple who have children with cystic fibrosis is 25%. These are population-based recurrence risks. If we were to study 1000 children born to parents with a dominant characteristic, we would not be surprised if the number of children with the dominant character was very close to 500, or 50%. On the other hand, if we study each child individually, we find a simple presence or absence of the character, that is, 0% or 100% risk. Population risks are obviously average risks.

In many cases, we can do better than the population-based risks and calculate a personal risk based upon specific evidence. When we speak of population risks, we really speak of a pool of gametes. When we try to calculate personal risks, we want to know the answer to the following question: of a pool of gametes with two possible genotypes, what was the genotype of the specific gamete that became you?

The type of evidence that is available to answer that question, either in whole or in part, depends upon what stage of the life cycle we are studying (gamete, zygote, chorionic villus sample [CVS], amniocytes, child, adult, etc.), whether the test is predictive or descriptive, whether the character that the test measures is expressed at that stage of personal development, and so forth.

As a general introduction, let us consider several types of evidence and the ways in which they can be used. In the following chapters, we will study each of these in depth. Unless stated to the contrary for specific examples, it is assumed throughout that we are trying to detect the carrier state (heterozygotes) rather than the affected state if the test is performed following birth and that we are trying to detect the affected state if a test is performed during pregnancy.

1.1   Mendelian Risk

The Mendelian risk is the same as the population-based risk discussed above and does not involve testing. The recurrence risk for dominant diseases is 50%, for recessive diseases it is 25%, and so forth. In the case of genes on the X or Y chromosomes, inheritance and expression will obviously also be influenced by sex. Straightforward Mendelian risks refer, of course, to the chance of inheriting the gene, which is not necessarily the same as developing the disease except when penetrance and expressivity are both complete. If incomplete penetrance or variable expressivity is a known phenomenon for that particular disease, population studies can often give reasonable empirical modification factors to the basic Mendelian risk.

Population risks are also used in a slightly different manner when someone who has a close relative with an autosomal recessive disease is concerned about the risk of having a child affected by the same disorder. For the partner with the family history, the risk is calculated based upon the degree of relationship to the closest obligate carrier. Assuming that the partner marrying into the family has no previous family history of that disease, the population frequency of heterozygotes must be determined. This is determined mathematically by use of the Hardy-Weinberg principle. Some diseases also have a considerable ethnic component that is very relevant to the determination of such risk, and for this reason, it is standard practice in genetic counseling to ask about ethnic origins.

1.2   Risk Modified by Reproductive History

The phrase "risk modified by reproductive history" refers to what we call Bayesian risk, which is most frequently applied to X-linked recessive conditions. Each son of a potential female carrier must inherit one of her two X chromosomes. The more times she "tests" an X chromosome by having sons, the more likely it is that both of her

X chromosomes will be represented among them. If the sons are all healthy, this increases the likelihood that neither of her X chromosomes carries the mutation and that she actually is not a carrier of the disease.

1.3   Risk Based upon Phenotype

Most biochemical tests and most clinical tests are tests of phenotypes. It is assumed that possession of a mutation in a particular gene will reveal itself in some manner that can be detected either in a biochemical assay or as a clinical characteristic. The identification of carriers of X-linked diseases is perhaps the greatest priority of these types of test because of the high risk of having an affected son. Examples of biochemical tests that can help to identify such carriers are clotting assays for the hemophilias, levels of muscle creatine kinase (CK M) in the blood for the muscular dystrophies, or very long chain fatty acids for adrenoleukodystrophy. Some carriers also experience mild symptoms of the disease and can be detected clinically (manifesting heterozygotes).

The identification of carriers of autosomal recessive conditions is usually less pressing because normally one carrier in the partnership is not sufficient to produce a child with the disease. This situation changes when their ethnic origins are known to be associated with markedly increased risk of both partners being carriers or when one partner has a positive family history of the disease. In such cases, if a screening test is available, there would be obvious benefit from its application.

The presymptomatic identification of heterozygotes for autosomal dominant diseases with delayed onset is also of considerable interest when the disease causes significant hardship or when the identification of such carriers can lead to early intervention and prophylactic therapy. Examples of this type of test are neurological examination for Huntington disease (for reproductive or lifestyle decisions), bowel examination for familial polyposis, or pentagastrin screening for multiple endocrine neoplasia type 2A. In the latter two examples, removal of the target organ where tumors will grow (colon or thyroid) when precancerous stages of the disease are detected can have great prophylactic value (risks for all three conditions can also be modified quite precisely through DNA analysis).

1.4   Risk Based upon Genotype

Predictive tests of genotypes are almost exclusively DNA-based tests. In the absence of DNA testing, it is difficult to predict a genotype unless there is genetic proof that no alternative exists. Rare examples of the latter occur when homozygotes reproduce, such as two people affected by the same type of recessive albinism or an individual homozygous for a dominant condition. When DNA testing is possible, the inheritance of a particular allele at the DNA test locus has direct predictive value for the inherited genotype at the linked disease-causing (or other) locus of interest. Since the event that determines the accuracy of DNA tests occurs during meiosis (in the previous generation), nothing that happens during one's own lifetime influences the predictive accuracy of these tests. In this sense, they are "black or white" tests: absolutely correct or absolutely wrong, depending solely upon whether or not a recombination event took place in the critical region in that particular meiosis. This is in marked contrast to phenotypic tests, the results of which may be modified by many factors (and which may therefore be considered to be equivalent to "shades of gray"). For instance, the assay of factor VIII levels (F8C) as a predictor of carrier status for hemophilia A may be influenced by many variables, including age, general health, medication (oral contraceptives), pregnancy, nonrandom X chromosome inactivation, and ABO blood type.

1.5   Familial versus New Mutations

Although all of the conditions addressed in this book are considered to be genetic, or, more specifically, heritable, the fact that a couple has a child affected with a single-gene hereditary disease caused by the mutation of a specific gene does not necessarily mean that one or both parents must also possess the mutation(s). It is perfectly possible, and sometimes quite common, for the first affected person in a family to have a new mutation that neither parent possessed. The mode of inheritance obviously is very significant in trying to determine the likelihood that an affected individual has a new mutation. A single affected individual in a family is called an isolated case. An isolated case with a fully penetrant dominant disease almost certainly has a new mutation; an isolated case with a common recessive disease is unlikely to have a new mutation (and extremely unlikely to have two new mutations). X-linked conditions tend to lie between these two extremes; the proportion of affected sons born to noncarrier mothers increases with the increasing genetic lethality of the condition.

1.6 Meiotic versus Mitotic Mutations

Mutations are caused by damage to DNA and/or by errors in the replication of DNA molecules. Only heritable mutations, those occurring in cell lines that might ultimately yield mutant gametes, are considered in this book; somatic mutations confined to a single generation are not considered, even though they cause a major fraction of human health problems. Since DNA must be replicated before each mitotic or meiotic division, mutations can occur in either process. If a mutation occurs in meiosis, the resultant gamete will contain a mutation not found in any cell of the parent. Two assumptions can be made: (*a*) the parent will be completely asymptomatic, since the parental genome does not possess the mutation, and (*b*) the recurrence risk is extremely low (equal to the probability of an independent mutation occurring within the same gene).

If the mutation occurs during mitosis, however, the two assumptions just stated no longer apply. Mutations that occur in a mitosis close to the end of the developmental process may appear to approximate meiotic mutations, since few cells in the parent's body will possess the mutation and perhaps a very restricted subpopulation of gametes will be mutant; mutations occurring in an earlier mitosis (such as early embryogenesis) may result in significant somatic symptoms and/or a high recurrence risk. A half-chromatid mutation in a sperm or ovum would represent an extreme example of this type of problem. The main difficulty in a diagnostic setting is to try to estimate where on this spectrum the case in hand falls.

1.7 Non-Mendelian Genetic Mechanisms

Because risk prediction for single-gene disorders generally assumes Mendelian inheritance, it is appropriate to include from the outset a list of potential circumstances where Mendelian assumptions might not apply. These should be taken very seriously and be remembered as potential disclaimers to the implicit assumption of Mendelian inheritance throughout the rest of this book.

Nonpaternity is included first in this list of potential problems: (*a*) because of its frequency and (*b*) because all risk predictions based upon linkage depend upon the source of marker alleles being that assumed from the given pedigree. There are other, presumably less frequent, mechanisms of nonparentage such as hospital mix-ups, unknown adoption, and elder siblings raising the illegitimate offspring of their younger siblings as their own. Nonparentage is not a problem (technically, at least) when the disease-causing mutation is known and the predictions have been based directly upon its inheritance or lack thereof. Null alleles can also mimic nonparentage in a DNA test, and although apparent nonmaternity tends to make us stop and think about possible unusual mechanisms, null alleles should at least be considered as an alternative to apparent nonpaternity (particularly for autosomal conditions when the father is not obviously heterozygous at that locus). In the opposite sense, when we are intentionally studying the question of family relationships, as in paternity studies, these considerations plus other mechanisms discussed below (disomy, in particular) mean that the inference of nonparentage should probably be based upon the noninheritance of loci on at least two different chromosomes. Uniparental disomy can also mimic nonparentage, by a different mechanism; in the case of null alleles, the parent donates an "invisible" allele, but chromosome segregation follows normal Mendelian inheritance; in the case of disomy, the parent really does fail to donate a copy of a particular chromosome (but does donate the other 22 chromosomes and is still the true parent). Uniparental disomy, therefore, is clearly a non-Mendelian mechanism.

In the absence of polymorphisms or disease-causing mutations, the base sequence of the alleles inherited from each parent should be the same. Even when this is so, the two alleles do not necessarily function equally: the maternal allele may be expressed to a greater extent than the paternal allele, or vice versa. The mechanism by which the expression of alleles can be modified for one generation is called *imprinting*. Alleles (or more likely whole chromosomal regions) are imprinted during meiosis; the imprint is maintained through multiple mitoses, and then erased, repeated, or reversed during the next meiosis (one generation later). The most likely mechanism of imprinting is through variation in the degree of methylation of bases. Parental differences had been documented for some time in rodents, in which it is possible, through the selective breeding of translocation carriers, to generate offspring that contain both regions of a given chromosome from the same parent. In humans, one of the key observations was that a small number of individuals affected with autosomal recessive conditions sometimes also had a very specific additional set of unusual characteristics (such as cystic fibrosis (CF) associated with small stature). The subsequent finding that only one of the two parents was a carrier of CF and/or that both copies of chromosome 7 could be shown to be derived from the same parent showed that unusual genetic mechanisms could perhaps explain the characteristics added to the basic syndrome. A second key observation was the demonstration through molecular genetics that some individuals with Prader-Willi syndrome or

Angelman syndrome, two clinically quite distinct entities, shared very similar deletions of part of chromosome 15, but the parental origin of such deletions (or the parental origin of the remaining functional chromosome) was different for the two syndromes (see review of imprinting by Hall, 1990).

Uniparental *disomy* means the inheritance of two copies of a chromosome from one parent (and, in an individual with 46 chromosomes, a lack of inheritance of that chromosome from the other parent). This has been identified in cases of well-known recessive diseases where there have also been additional unusual phenotypic characteristics not normally associated with that disease (such as cystic fibrosis combined with short stature). It has also been associated with cases of diseases where imprinting plays a significant role (such as Prader-Willi syndrome) because the lack of contribution from one parent will cause an obvious imbalance in chromosomal imprinting. In the case of recessive diseases, two like copies of a particular chromosome are inherited from the same parent (uniparental homodisomy or isodisomy); the inheritance of the two different copies of a particular chromosome (uniparental heterodisomy) would generate carrier offspring for autosomal recessive disorders. Either homodisomy or heterodisomy might lead to the expression of the abnormality when that region of the genome should have been specifically imprinted by the parent who failed to contribute a copy of that chromosome. It is actually very difficult to keep descriptions of the mechanisms leading to clinical disorders technically correct. The foregoing statements about recessive diseases really pertain to specific loci on chromosomes, whereas disomy pertains to chromosomes. Recombination can make the interpretation of the origin of specific alleles and loci quite difficult; discussion of this will be saved for section 7.6. Since uniparental heterodisomy might well be without phenotypic consequence when specific imprinting of that region of the genome is not mandatory, a study of its frequency in the general population is needed because of its implications for the segregation of alleles in linkage analyses and its consequences for risk predictions based upon the assumed "Mendelian" segregation of alleles. Paternal heterodisomy involving both the X and Y chromosome has accounted for at least one instance of the transmission of hemophilia A from a 46,XY father to a 46,XY son.

Gene conversion is a phenomenon arising from faulty correction of mismatched DNA strands. Although it is difficult to study in human populations, it is known to occur, and the major consequence of gene conversion to risk prediction would be its ability to mimic a meiotic double crossover in a (potentially extremely) confined stretch of DNA. Laboratories that study diseases that seem to involve either recombination anomalies or erratic "hot spots" of recombination very close to the disease locus should keep this mechanism in mind. Similarly, it should be kept in mind as an alternative explanation for an "impossible" double crossover.

When we discuss human embryogenesis, we normally assume that one fertilized ovum will eventually develop into one complete human. Not all pregnancies follow this assumption. *Monozygotic twinning* splits a single mass of cells into two (or more) separate embryos (conceptually one human in two bodies). *Chimerism,* on the other hand, fuses two separate embryos into one (conceptually two different humans in one body). Twinning is obvious, and its frequency is known with considerable accuracy. Chimerism may be extremely rare, or it may be more common than we think because it might escape detection (after all, there is nothing abnormal about giving birth to a single baby). Same-sex chimerism might be a potential alternative explanation for what appears to be somatic mosaicism.

Why worry about either of these? There are several reports of female monozygotic twins who are discordant for the expression of X-linked diseases. One of the steps leading to monozygotic twinning might be the accumulation of concentrations of cells that have the same inactivated X chromosome at opposite poles of the developing cell mass. If this is so, monozygotic female twins who were also carriers of an X-linked disorder would be expected to be discordant to the extent that one of them is symptomatic. Since monozygotic twinning occurs in approximately 1 in 200 pregnancies, it is perhaps relevant to consider the possibility that female "carriers" identified by prenatal diagnosis might be symptomatic by this mechanism. Cases of skewed Lyonization in single births might also be encompassed by this mechanism if there had been a twin at an early stage in the pregnancy who died and was absorbed.

Some very interesting hypotheses have been put forward by Gil Côté which warrant consideration here (Côté 1989a, 1989b; Côté and Gyftodimou 1991). These hypotheses propose that *cis-trans effects* resulting from meiotic or mitotic crossing-over are involved in many instances where diseases do not conform to the basic Mendelian ratios. I cannot do justice to the far-reaching consequences of these hypotheses in a short review, but as an example, if there are two linked loci with alleles A and B at one and R and S at the other, these will be inherited in the same configuration as the parental haplotypes unless recombination occurs between them. If only one haplotype, say B-R, causes disease when the B and R are in a *cis*-configuration (on the same chromosome), an individual with A-R/B-S haplotypes would be unaffected, whereas an individual with the same alleles in the opposite configuration, A-S/B-R, would be affected (if B-R causes a dominant disease). Meiotic recombination between these two linked loci might explain pedigrees with nonpenetrance (and particularly the more unusual pedigrees where distant relatives are connected through many apparently normal individuals). The rate of "reversion" should be about the same, and penetrant individuals might be expected to have nonpenetrant children who nevertheless carry the components of the "mutation." Mitotic recombination might explain widely differing expressivity. As one last example, mitotic crossing-over before monozygotic twinning may disrupt genomic imprinting as well as the *cis*-acting combinations described above. More important, however, are the possibilities that (*a*) mitotic crossing-over might actually induce twinning, and (*b*) that "crossed" X chromosomes might be unable to be inactivated. If this is so, mitotic crossing-over in female embryos carrying mutations for X-linked diseases might not only increase the likelihood of forming monozygotic female twins but also ensure that one of them will be affected with the disease.

In traditional Mendelian genetics it is generally assumed that mutations "breed true," that is, with the exception of variable expressivity in autosomal dominant conditions, the symptoms experienced by one affected individual are generally a good prediction of what can be expected in the next. One does not normally find mild hemophilia and severe hemophilia in different members of the same family. In the case of variable expressivity, the genotype is very predictable even if the phenotype is not. It is becoming increasingly apparent that there are regions of *genomic instability* that are predisposed to undergo major mutation within the span of a single generation. This predisposition is sometimes referred to as a "premutation," meaning that although the person carrying it has few or no phenotypic consequences, when that person reproduces, there is a potential to convert the premutation into a "full" mutation and have an affected child. Furthermore, since the region can undergo major mutation between one generation and the next, there may be an unpredictable extent to which it mutates. At present, fragile X syndrome, Kennedy disease (spinal and bulbar muscular atrophy), and myotonic dystrophy are the best known examples of diseases in which unstable regions can show progressive degenerative changes between different generations. It is very likely that further unstable regions will be demonstrated, associated with other diseases that show a progression in severity of symptoms through the generations (anticipation). As a general rule, the possibility of back-mutation from mutant to normal can be ignored in human genetics. In the case of these unstable regions, at least a theoretical mechanism exists by which mutant genotypes could revert to normal. This phenomenon has been described in fragile X syndrome and myotonic dystrophy but does not appear to happen to any useful extent, based upon the limited information available at the time of writing. If any diseases are identified where unequal crossing-over is shown to be the cause of the instability, however, the prospects of back-mutation would be better (studies with flanking DNA markers in fragile X syndrome and myotonic dystrophy have ruled out unequal single crossovers as the mechanism for mutation).

Last but certainly not least, we must consider *mitochondrial inheritance*. Mitochondria contain a circular DNA molecule that encodes mitochondrial ribosomal RNA and some of the components of the respiratory chain. According to the endosymbiont theory, an ancient progenitor of the mitochondrion was an independent bacterial-type cell. Following its capture by an ancient progenitor of the modern eukaryotic cell, it has undergone what amounts to a systematic and progressive enslavement process. Significant in the genetic sense is the fact that perhaps because it is somewhat sheltered from selective pressures by being inside a stable cellular environment, the mitochondrial DNA mutates at a much faster rate than our nuclear DNA. Mitochondria and mitochondrial DNA are also inherited only from the ovum, giving a purely matrilineal mechanism of inheritance. All cells in our body contain a very large number of mitochondria and, therefore, also a very large number of mitochondrial chromosomes (up to many thousands).

Mitochondria divide by binary fission and are apportioned randomly between the new cells following nuclear division during mitosis or meiosis. What is the significance of all this to mutations of mitochondrial DNA? First, mitochondrial mutations show maternal transmission only. Second, the degree of expression of symptoms may be highly variable because the relative proportions of normal and abnormal mitochondria may vary significantly not only from sibling to sibling but also between regions of the same body and even between adjacent cells originally derived from a common progenitor (most cells would be heteroplasmic). Therefore, although all children of an affected mother should be affected, it is usually not possible to predict how affected they will be. Such predictions would be easy if we knew that the mother possessed 100% mutant mitochondria (homoplasmic), but this state is certain to be extremely rare if not impossible.

As an example, let us assume that the cells in a woman's ovaries that will give rise to her ova contain an average of 80% mutant and 20% normal mitochondrial DNA. To obtain this overall proportion, individual cells might be 50:50, 90:10, 81:19, etc. The risk to each child will depend upon which exact progenitor cell produced the ovum, the ratio of mutant to normal mitochondria in the ovum, how the mito-chondria segregate following fertilization and during development, and what ratios of mutant to normal mitochondria are required for clinical/subclinical expression. Finally, we are starting to obtain evidence in humans of a phenomenon that has been known for a long time in other eukaryotic organisms, namely, for some types of mitochondrial mutation, the relative proportions of mutant and normal mitochondria change significantly over time even within the same cell and such a change may be in one direction only (usually in favor of normal) or may be periodic or cyclical.

Having taken some trouble to emphasize some of the potential "dis-claimers," I will discuss in the following chapters various ways of estimating genetic risks in depth (assuming conventional Mendelian inheritance unless otherwise specified).

2

Bayesian Risk Calculations

for X-Linked Recessive Disorders

The guiding principle behind Bayesian calculations is to consider the likelihood of two or more alternative hypotheses, given a set of known conditions or results. In human genetics, the contrasting hypotheses usually take the form of the probability that someone has or has not inherited a disease-causing allele of a gene. In Figure 2.1, there are four families. In each family, assume that the female in the second generation is the daughter of an obligate carrier of an X-linked recessive disorder.

2.1 Unaffected Sons

As shown in Figure 2.1, in family A, the daughter has no children; in family B, she has one normal son; in family C, two normal sons; and in family D, three normal sons. At birth, she had a 50% risk of being a carrier. This is called her *prior probability* and represents the probability that she inherited the mutant allele from her mother in the absence of consideration of any other evidence. The basic logic behind Bayesian calculations is that if she is a carrier, there would be a 50% chance of passing on the mutant allele to each child or, conversely, a 50% chance of passing on the normal allele. These are *conditional probabilities* because they are the chance, for each hypothesis, of a given condition occurring if that hypothesis is correct. The conditional probability of having a normal son if she is a carrier is 0.5. Note also that the conditional probabilities are different for the different hypotheses. If she is not a carrier, the chance that a son would be

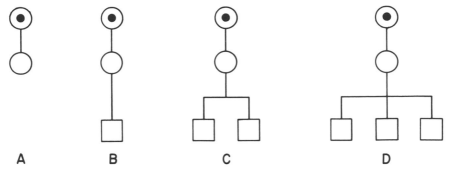

Figure 2.1   A series of families in which the female in the first generation of each family is an obligate carrier of an X-linked recessive disorder. In each family, she has a daughter and 0 to 3 normal grandsons. The daughter might be a carrier of the disease. Tables 2.1 and 2.2 show how different numbers of normal grandsons alter the risk that the daughter is a carrier.

normal is no longer 50%; it is 100%, because it no longer matters which X chromosome the son inherits when both are normal. Since the conditional probabilities usually represent independent events (in family D, three independent pregnancies), they are multiplied together. The *joint probability* is the product of the prior probability multiplied by all the conditional probabilities. Comparison of the magnitude of the joint probabilities tells us something about the relative likelihood of our original hypotheses.

The steps are very simple (Table 2.1). The hypotheses are written out side by side and the mathematics pertaining to each hypothesis is filled in below it, so two (or more) columns of numbers are generated. For family D, the two hypotheses are that the female, II-1, is a carrier or is a noncarrier. Below this is written the prior probability of each hypothesis, then the conditional probabilities (that son 1 is normal, that son 2 is normal, etc.) for each hypothesis.

Note that the joint probabilities (0.0625 and 0.5) do not add up to 1.0, so they cannot be directly converted to percentages. These are frequently converted to *posterior probabilities* out of 1.0 (normalized) by the following step. The posterior probability for each column is its joint probability divided by the sum of the joint probabilities of all columns. Here 0.0625 divided by 0.0625 + 0.5 (or 0.5625) = 0.1111. Likewise, 0.5/(0.0625 + 0.5) = 0.8889. These are directly convertible to percentages (11.11% and 88.89%). Taking into account the fact that this female has three normal sons who each had an equal chance of inheriting the mutant allele if she were a carrier has reduced the risk that she is a carrier from her prior risk of 50% to her posterior risk of

Table 2.1   Calculation for family D in Figure 2.1

	Carrier	Noncarrier
Prior probability	0.5	0.5
Conditional probabilities		
that son 1 is normal	0.5	1.0
that son 2 is normal	0.5	1.0
that son 3 is normal	0.5	1.0
Joint probability	0.0625	0.5 (Total = 0.5625)
Posterior probability	0.0625/0.5625 = 0.1111	0.5000/0.5625 = 0.8889

about 11%. Similar calculations can be performed for each of the other families in Figure 2.1. Family A has no events to consider as conditional probabilities, family B has one event (the conditional probability of having one normal son), and family C has two independent events. The calculations for all four families are developed in parallel in Table 2.2.

This series of calculations provides a mathematical description of something that should be intuitively obvious: the more events that took place that could have identified the female as being a carrier if she were one, but that failed to do so, the less likely it is that she actually is a carrier. If she were a carrier, the more sons she had, the more likely it would be that at least one would have inherited the mutant allele and would manifest the disease. Although in this example we have considered something that can be tested biologically with complete certainty, that is, if a son inherits the mutant allele from a carrier mother he will be affected, the same logic will be used later in situations where the same rules of nature apply but we cannot directly see the consequences of a person's inheritance.

The more mathematically inclined reader will have noted that there is a direct relationship between the number of unaffected sons and the posterior risk of being a carrier. If the joint probabilities were expressed as fractions rather than decimal numbers, they would be $\frac{1}{2}$, $\frac{1}{4}$, $\frac{1}{8}$, and $\frac{1}{16}$ in the carrier column and always $\frac{1}{2}$ in the noncarrier column, which, when expressed as ratios between the two columns, become 1:1, 1:2, 1:4, and 1:8. In other words, the posterior risk is 1 out of 2, 3, 5, or 9, respectively. The general formula for the posterior risk with N unaffected sons when the prior risk was 0.5 is therefore $1/([2^N] + 1)$.

In some tables I have used decimals and in other tables I have used fractions. Many people will have learned the rudiments of Bayesian

Table 2.2   Calculations for all families in Figure 2.1

	Family A		Family B		Family C		Family D	
	C	NC	C	NC	C	NC	C	NC
Prior probability	0.5	0.5	0.5	0.5	0.5	0.5	0.5	0.5
Conditional probabilities								
that son 1 is normal			0.5	1.0	0.5	1.0	0.5	1.0
that son 2 is normal					0.5	1.0	0.5	1.0
that son 3 is normal							0.5	1.0
Joint probability	0.5	0.5	0.25	0.5	0.125	0.5	0.0625	0.5
Posterior probability	0.500	0.500	0.333	0.667	0.200	0.800	0.111	0.889
	(50%)		(33%)		(20%)		(11%)	

Note: C − carrier, NC = noncarrier.

calculations using fractions. On the other hand, the use of decimals is clearly more modern, and decimals will be used almost exclusively when dealing with DNA tests. I think that it is a good idea to be able to perform calculations both ways, although I have tended to favor decimals in this book except under specific circumstances. The use of decimals is very prone to the introduction of rounding errors, particularly in long calculations; the use of fractions is not prone to this error and therefore is superior in some situations. It really does not matter which system you prefer as long as when using decimals, you do not round up until the final answer.

2.2   Daughters with Unaffected Grandsons

Because females have two X chromosomes, their phenotypes for an X-linked recessive disorder are not automatically indicative of their genotypes. A daughter with no external indication of her carrier status is generally ignored in determining the posterior risk of her mother. If the daughter has unaffected sons, however, then the same argument as above applies: if she is a carrier, she has had a chance to show it. The more sons she has, the more times a test of one of her X chromosomes is carried out. It follows that if she has an infinite number of unaffected sons, she cannot be a carrier. If she is an obligate noncarrier, she should count as strongly as her unaffected brother would in considering the posterior risk of her mother. The range of values that should be entered as a conditional probability for her mother starts at

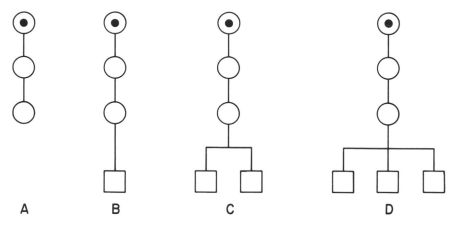

Figure 2.2   A series of families in which the female in the first generation of each family is an obligate carrier of an X-linked recessive disorder. In each family, she has a daughter, a granddaughter, and 0 to 3 normal great-grandsons. The daughter and the granddaughter might be carriers of the disease. Table 2.3 shows how the presence of the granddaughter with different numbers of normal great-grandsons alters the risk that the daughter is a carrier.

1.0 if she has no evidence to indicate noncarrier status and tends toward a minimum value of 0.5 with increasing evidence of her noncarrier status. If this value ever reaches 0.5, she must be an obligate noncarrier, since she now carries the same weight as her unaffected brother in whom there is a perfect correlation between genotype and phenotype.

Figure 2.2 adds an extra generation to the families in Figure 2.1. In this case, the consultand in the second generation has a daughter and a variable number of unaffected grandsons, and we are interested in determining the amount by which her daughter and her daughter's descendants modify her risk of being a carrier. The conditional probability of a daughter plus N unaffected grandsons is really identical to a miniature Bayesian calculation within the larger one for her mother (Table 2.3). The value entered into her mother's calculation is the sum of the two joint probabilities that would be obtained if the daughter was considered in isolation. The value is of the form $(P * Q^N) + (R * S^N)$, where P and R are the prior risks of her being a carrier or a noncarrier, respectively; if her mother is a carrier, $P = R = 0.5$. Q is the probability of each son's being unaffected if she is a carrier, raised to the power of the number of sons (0.5^N); S is the probability of each son's being unaffected if she is not a carrier, raised to the power N (1.0^N). The two joint probabilities are added, since they are not independent; if she is a carrier, she cannot be a noncarrier as well.

Table 2.3 Calculation of the conditional probabilities that the second-generation female in Figure 2.2 would have a daughter with *N* unaffected grandsons if she is a carrier

	Carrier	Noncarrier	Total
Family A no grandson	$(\frac{1}{2} * \frac{1}{2}^0)$ +	$(\frac{1}{2} * 1^0)$	$= 1/2 + 1/2 = 1$
Family B 1 grandson	$(\frac{1}{2} * \frac{1}{2}^1)$ +	$(\frac{1}{2} * 1^1)$	$= 1/4 + 1/2 = 3/4$
Family C 2 grandsons	$(\frac{1}{2} * \frac{1}{2}^2)$ +	$(\frac{1}{2} * 1^2)$	$= 1/8 + 1/2 = 5/8$
Family D 3 grandsons	$(\frac{1}{2} * \frac{1}{2}^3)$ +	$(\frac{1}{2} * 1^3)$	$= 1/16 + 1/2 = 9/16$

Note: Any number raised to the power $0 = 1$.

Table 2.4 Values to be entered into the conditional probability column for the mother

N	*N* Unaffected Sons		Daughters with *N* Unaffected Grandsons	
	Decimal	Fraction	Decimal	Fraction
0	1.0000	1/1	1.0000	2/2
1	0.5000	1/2	0.7500	3/4
2	0.2500	1/4	0.6250	5/8
3	0.1250	1/8	0.5625	9/16
4	0.0625	1/16	0.53125	17/32
5	0.03125	1/32	0.515625	33/64
6	0.015625	1/64	0.5078125	65/128
7	0.0078125	1/128	0.5039063	129/256
8	0.0039063	1/256	0.5019531	257/512
9	0.0019531	1/512	0.5009766	513/1024
10	0.0009766	1/1024	0.5004883	1025/2048
N	0.5^N	$1/2^N$	$[0.5(0.5)^N] + [0.5(1.0)^N]$	$(2^N + 1)/2^{N+1}$

Table 2.4 gives the conditional probability values for 0 to 10 unaffected sons and for a daughter with 0 to 10 unaffected grandsons.

2.3 Which Branches of the Family May Be Used?

The next important principle in performing Bayesian calculations is to know for each person which relatives can legitimately be used for conditional probability calculations. The reason for considering eligibility is to avoid circular arguments in which a daughter or her descen-

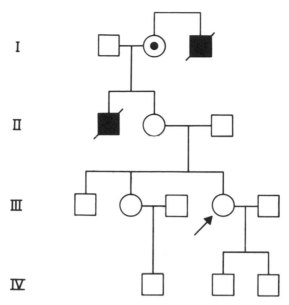

Figure 2.3   A family with an X-linked recessive disease. Tables 2.5 and 2.6 show
the steps Involved in the calculation of the risk that female III-4 is a carrier.

dants are used to modify the mother's risk to generate a posterior risk
that will then be applied to the daughter. This allows the daughter to
reduce her own prior risk, which will inevitably reduce her posterior
risk. If the daughter has a lower posterior risk, this could then be used
to modify her mother's risk again, and so on ad infinitum. This is
clearly not a legitimate process. The steps to follow so that the arguments are noncircular are (1) start with the earliest person of unknown
genotype; (2) use all branches of this person's family except the consul-
tant's branch to modify her risk; (3) halve her posterior risk to obtain
the prior risk for the next female down the consultand's branch; (4)
continue steps 2 and 3 until the consultand is reached and her prior
risk determined; and (5) use any of her descendants to obtain her
posterior risk.

   Figure 2.3 shows a family in which the consultand III-4 has a brother
and a sister/nephew combination who could modify her mother's carrier risk, as well as two sons of her own to modify the prior risk that
she inherited from her mother. Following the steps listed above, we
see that the earliest person of unknown genotype is the consultand's
mother, II-2, who has a prior risk of 50% of being a carrier (Table 2.5).

Table 2.5   Calculation of a provisional posterior risk for II-2 in Figure 2.3 for use
in the calculation of her daughter's risk

	Carrier	Noncarrier
Prior probability	1/2	1/2
Conditional probabilities		
III-1	1/2	1
III-2 and IV-1	3/4	1
Joint probability	3/16	1/2 or 8/16 (Total = 11/16)
Posterior probability	3/11	8/11

Table 2.6   Calculation of the risk for III-4 in Figure 2.3

	Carrier	Noncarrier
Prior probability	3/22	19/22
Conditional probabilities		
that IV-2 is normal	1/2	1
that IV-3 is normal	1/2	1
Joint probability	3/88	19/22 or 76/88 (Total = 79/88)
Posterior probability	3/79	76/79

The consultand's brother, III-1, counts as a factor of $\frac{1}{2}$ in the conditional probability column for her mother, and the consultand's sister with the nephew counts as a factor of $\frac{3}{4}$ (see Table 2.4).

The prior risk for consultand III-4 is therefore $\frac{3}{22}$, and her posterior risk is this modified by her two unaffected sons (Table 2.6). If the consultand had a daughter, her prior risk would be $\frac{3}{158}$. Note that if III-2 were the consultand instead of III-4, the posterior risk for their mother, II-2, would be different, since the conditional probability of $\frac{3}{4}$ used for III-2 would now be replaced by $\frac{5}{8}$ (two sons) for III-4. Finally, if the mother II-2 were the consultand, both daughters could be used as conditional probabilities for her.

As a final, rather obvious point, the mode of inheritance always overrules mathematical risk calculations. If a female is an obligate carrier of a disease, normal sons are a blessing but cannot be used in a Bayesian calculation to reduce her risk. (However, they do affect the overall probability of the pedigree as calculated by computer programs, and they may contribute significantly to gene-mapping studies.)

2.4 Negative Family History

In the preceding section, we considered cases where the mother of the consultand has either been an obligate carrier or had a known risk of being a carrier because of her descent from one. When the family has only one male affected with the disease, the possibility that he has a new mutation must be considered, because if this is so, his mother is not a carrier. Similarly, his mother may be a carrier but have a new mutation herself, in which case only she has any danger of having more affected children. In this section, therefore, there is an additional question to be answered in considering the difference between familial and isolated cases. The question has two parts: (*a*) is this a new mutation? and (*b*) if so, in which generation did it occur? The mechanics of how we approach such families are different: previously, we studied the relationship between the consultand and the last obligate carrier ancestral to her and any evidence that suggests that the carrier may or may not have passed the mutation down to the consultand; in considering an isolated case, we must study the relationship between the consultand and the mother of the affected male and any evidence to suggest that the consultand might have inherited the mutation. Whereas the former almost always starts at the top of the pedigree and works down, the latter may do the same, or start at the bottom and work up, or both. We also need two additional pieces of information that did not apply to familial cases.

(1) We need to know the reproductive fitness (*f*) of males affected with the disease. Fitness is a measure of the ability of affected individuals to pass on their genotype; it should not be confused with longevity. If the individual is sterile, is physically or mentally unable to reproduce, or invariably dies before reproducing, his fitness is 0 (as in Duchenne muscular dystrophy); if affected males reproduce as successfully as their unaffected brothers, the fitness is 1.0 (as in protan/deutan color blindness). Many X-linked diseases have fitness values (*f*) between 0 and 1. If the fitness is greater than 0, there is a possibility that, in unknown relatives in former generations, the disease may have been passed through males as well as females, giving an increased number of theoretical sources of the disease found in our contemporary proband.

(2) We need to know the mutation rate, or, more specifically, the sex-specific mutation rates, if they are different. The female mutation rate is denoted by the symbol μ (Greek letter mu), and the male mutation rate is denoted by the symbol ν (Greek letter nu). If the rates are the same, or different but unknown and therefore treated as the same out of ignorance, they are both labeled μ. (Since mutation rates can

be calculated in many different ways, it is also necessary to know the units.)

There are formal mathematical proofs of carrier risks for mothers of isolated cases. I will present here only a simple logical argument instead of the more complex mathematical methods (which are nevertheless in agreement). Consider a female who has a son affected with Duchenne muscular dystrophy ($f = 0$) and who has no known family history of that disease. Several possibilities exist: her son could have a new mutation, she could be a carrier of a mutation that was new in her, her mother could be a carrier of a new mutation, her grandmother could be a carrier of a new mutation, etc. Of all these possibilities, she is a noncarrier only when her son has a new mutation. Since she has two X chromosomes, she would be a carrier is she inherited a new mutation on her paternal X chromosome (v) or if she inherited an existing mutation on her maternal X chromosome (half of her mother's carrier risk) or a new mutation on her maternal X chromosome (μ). If we treat the male and female mutation rates as equal (both represented by μ), each female has a risk equal to half of her mother's risk plus an additional 2μ. Since $f = 0$, there is no possibility of the disease having been passed through an affected male. This leads to the formulation of an infinite series, where

$$\text{Risk} = 2\mu + \tfrac{1}{2}(2\mu) + \tfrac{1}{4}(2\mu) + \tfrac{1}{8}(2\mu), \text{ etc.}$$

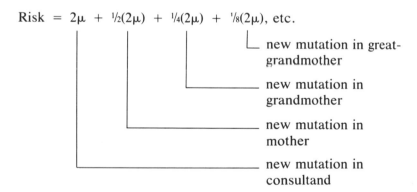

new mutation in great-grandmother

new mutation in grandmother

new mutation in mother

new mutation in consultand

The multipliers of $\tfrac{1}{2}$, $\tfrac{1}{4}$, $\tfrac{1}{8}$, etc., refer to the probability of inheriting the mutation from that person through the intervening number of generations. This series can be rearranged by placing the 2μ outside the brackets to obtain $2\mu (1 + \tfrac{1}{2} + \tfrac{1}{4} + \tfrac{1}{8} + \dots)$, which (after an infinite number of generations) will eventually become $2\mu(2)$, or 4μ. This is the (population) risk that any female with a negative family history of Duchenne muscular dystrophy is a carrier of the disease, expressed as a multiple of the mutation rate. To obtain the carrier risk when she has an affected son requires a Bayesian calculation to

Figure 2.4   A small family where the affected son is the only known person (isolated case) affected by an X-linked recessive disease that is genetically lethal (affected individuals cannot reproduce). Since he is the only known affected individual, his mother is not necessarily a carrier. Her risk is calculated in Table 2.7.

Table 2.7   Calculation for the mother of an isolated case

	Carrier	Noncarrier
Prior probability	4μ	$1 - 4\mu \approx 1$
Conditional probabilities		
affected son	$0.5 + \mu \approx 0.5$†	μ
Joint probability	2μ	μ
Posterior probability	0.667	0.333

† From this point onward, I will ignore μ in terms like $1 - 4\mu$ or $0.5 + \mu$ (mutation of gametes) or $0.5 (1 + \mu)$ (mutation before gametogenesis), since μ is trivial in comparison to numbers within an order of magnitude of unity.

determine the probability of his having the disease under the opposing conditions of her being either a carrier or a noncarrier (Figure 2.4 and Table 2.7).

From this point onward, I will ignore μ in expressions such as $1 - 4\mu$ or $0.5 + \mu$, since μ is trivial in comparison to the other number. The absolute value of μ is usually less than $1/10{,}000$. Computer programs do not ignore these small numbers and may show slightly different results.

The conclusion from this calculation is that for an X-linked genetically lethal disease, when the male and female mutation rates are equal, the mother of an isolated case, in the absence of any other pedigree evidence, has a risk of $2/3$ of being a carrier of the disease. To reverse the emphasis, only $1/3$ of isolated affected males have noncarrier mothers and are the direct result of a new mutation. If the male and female mutation rates are not equal, then the formula $2\mu + 2\nu$ will give the population risk when both μ and ν are known and $f = 0$ (see Bundey 1978 for examples).

Note that as in the earlier discussion of familial cases the value of 0.5 is entered in the carrier column as the conditional probability; however, in this case, it is the probability of having an affected son, whereas previously it was the probability of having a normal son. Although this might seem odd at first, the value in the noncarrier column makes the big difference between the calculations for familial and isolated cases. In familial cases, the conditional probability entered in the noncarrier column of having a normal son is 1; in isolated cases, the probability entered in the noncarrier column of having an affected son is μ. The important factor for conditional probabilities is not the magnitude of the numbers used but rather the ratio between the columns. In the familial case, the numbers are 0.5 and 1.0, which have a ratio of 1:2 favoring noncarrier status; in the isolated case, the numbers are 0.5 and μ, which very strongly favors carrier status (μ is generally of the magnitude 10^{-5} or 10^{-6}), with a ratio of hundreds of thousands or millions to one. In the latter case, this is almost counteracted by the enormous ratio of the prior probabilities in the opposite direction ($4\mu:1$).

If the mother of the isolated case has other pedigree evidence that could bear upon her carrier status, it is included in the same manner as in the section on familial cases. For instance, if she also has a normal son, he can be used to reduce her carrier risk, as before (Figure 2.5 and Table 2.8).

For diseases that are not always genetically lethal, the fitness of affected males will be somewhere between 0 and 1. When there is the possibility that the disease might be passed through an affected male, the infinite series (used earlier to show that the population risk for any female to be a carrier of Duchenne muscular dystrophy was 4μ) no longer applies. Instead, each term following the initial 2μ for new mutations on her two X chromosomes now needs to have an additional factor to account for the possibility of the disease being passed through her father, maternal grandfather, maternal great-grandfather, paternal great-grandfather via paternal grandmother, etc. Remember also that if the male and female mutation rates are known to be different, it is necessary to be even more specific in deriving this very complex series of possibilities. Fortunately, none of this is necessary, since these problems were solved decades ago and the following, useful formulae are available:

$$C = (2 + f)/3 \qquad \text{(assuming } \mu = v) \qquad (2.1)$$
$$P = (1 - f)\mu/(2\mu + v) \qquad\qquad\qquad\quad (2.2a)$$
$$P = (1 - f)/3 \qquad \text{(assuming } \mu = v) \qquad (2.2b)$$
$$R = (1 - f)X/3, \text{ or } X = 3R/(1 - f) \qquad (2.3)$$

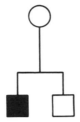

Figure 2.5   A small family similar to the family shown in Fig. 2.4 except that the mother of the isolated case has an additional son. His presence (slightly) reduces the probability that the mother is a carrier, as shown in Table 2.8.

Table 2.8   Calculation for Figure 2.5

	Carrier	Noncarrier
Prior probability	4μ	1
Conditional probabilities		
affected son	0.5	μ
normal son	0.5	1
Joint probability	μ	μ
Posterior probability	0.5	0.5

where C = proportion of mothers of isolated cases who are carriers;

P = proportion of affected males who are new mutants $(P + C = 1.0)$;

R = mutation rate assuming $\mu - \nu$; and

X = frequency of affected males.

To these we can add the following useful relationships:

$$N = (4 + 2f)/(1 - f) \qquad \text{(assuming } \mu = \nu) \qquad (2.4)$$
$$Y = 3/(1 - f) \qquad\qquad \text{(assuming } \mu = \nu) \qquad (2.5)$$

where N = coefficient of μ for the population frequency of female carriers (e.g., when $f = 0$ or 0.7, $N = 4$ or 18, respectively).

Y = coefficient of μ for the population frequency of affected males (e.g., when $f = 0$ or 0.7, $Y = 3$ or 10, respectively).

It is worth noting that there are formulae related to equation 2.3 (X – linked recessive) which give the mutation rates for autosomal diseases. (For autosomal diseases, X would be the frequency of affected individuals of either gender.)

$$R = (1 - f)X/2 \text{ for autosomal dominant diseases, and}$$
$$R = (1 - f)X \text{ for autosomal recessive diseases.}$$

Equation 2.4 is derived as follows. This derivation assumes that the population is in genetic equilibrium in the sense that the carrier risk of a daughter is the same as the carrier risk of her mother, and vice versa (e.g., all 4μ or all 18μ). Since it is a population-based calculation, we also have to take into consideration the possibility that her father might be affected. F is used for the frequency of female carriers and M for the frequency of affected males. Any female can be a carrier through the possession of a mutation coming from four different sources: (a) her mother was a carrier (probability F), in which case, her risk from this source is $F/2$; (b) a new mutation from her mother, risk μ; (c) her father was affected (probability M) and passed on the mutation, risk Mf; and (d) by new mutation from a normal father, risk ν. Since we are assuming that the population is in equilibrium, the sum of these four components will equal the population risk for her mother, F (i.e., the overall risk remains constant through the generations). The formula representing this equilibrium is therefore

$$F = F/2 + \mu + Mf + \nu$$

Finally, the probability of a male's being affected, M, can be derived from the probability that his mother was a carrier, F, plus the probability of a new mutation from a noncarrier mother, μ. Therefore, $M = F/2 + \mu$; f is the proportion of these mutations not lost from the population. Substituting this into the above expression, we obtain

$$F = F/2 + \mu + f(F/2 + \mu) + \nu$$
$$F/2 = \mu + fF/2 + f\mu + \nu$$
$$F/2 - fF/2 = \mu + f\mu + \nu$$
$$F/2 \, (1 - f) = \mu + f\mu + \nu$$
$$F = (2\mu + 2f\mu + 2\nu)/(1 - f) \tag{2.6}$$

If $\mu = \nu$, then F can be expressed as a multiple, N, of μ

$$N\mu = (4\mu + 2f\mu)/(1 - f)$$
$$N = (4 + 2f)/(1 - f) \tag{2.4}$$

If μ and ν are not equal, we must use equation 2.6 instead.

From the above collection of formulae we can derive all of the population statistics that we will commonly need. For example, if the fitness of males with hemophilia A averages 0.7, then $(2 + 0.7)/3$ or 0.9 (90%)

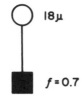

18μ

f = 0.7

Figure 2.6 A small family with an isolated case of an X-linked recessive disease which is not genetically lethal. In this case, affected males have a reproductive fitness (f) of 0.7. The probability that his mother is a carrier of the disease is calculated in Table 2.9.

Table 2.9   Calculation of the carrier risk for the mother of an isolated case of a disease that is not genetically lethal ($f = 0.7$)

	Carrier	Noncarrier
Prior probability	18μ†	1
Conditional probabilities		
affected son	0.5	μ
Joint probability	9μ	μ
Posterior probability	0.9	0.1

†The prior risk of 18μ when $f = 0.7$ is derived from equation 2.4 or can be obtained from Table 2.10.

will be the proportion of mothers of isolated cases who will be carriers (equation 2.1). This can also be approached from the perspective of finding out the population risk of any female to be a carrier of hemophilia A (18μ; $N = 18$ when $f = 0.7$; equation 2.4) and then deriving the carrier risk of such a female with an affected son by a Bayesian calculation similar to the one given previously for Duchenne muscular dystrophy (Figure 2.6 and Table 2.9).

Table 2.10 gives the posterior carrier risks for the mothers of isolated affected roles of several different values of f when the male and female mutation rates are equal ($\mu = \nu$). The interpretation of Table 2.10 is that if fitness $= 0.4$, the mother of an isolated affected male has an 80% risk of being a carrier in the absence of any information that might modify this risk. Table A.4 in the Appendix gives the posterior risk for the mother of an isolated affected male ($f = 0$) when she also has 0 to 5 normal brothers and 0 to 5 normal sons. Table A.5 shows the derivation of a general formula that will permit the calculation of similar results when $f > 0$.

Table 2.10 Posterior risks for mothers of isolated cases when $\mu = \nu$

		Posterior Risk	
f	Prior Risk	Carrier	Noncarrier
0	4μ	0.667	0.333
0.1	4.67μ	0.700	0.300
0.2	5.5μ	0.733	0.267
0.3	6.57μ	0.767	0.233
0.4	8μ	0.800	0.200
0.5	10μ	0.833	0.167
0.6	13μ	0.867	0.133
0.7	18μ	0.900	0.100
0.8	28μ	0.933	0.067
0.9	58μ	0.967	0.033
Column 1	2	3	4

When a significant fraction of cases of a disease are caused by new mutation (fitness is low), there is an approximate correlation between the size of the coding region of any given gene and the frequency with which affected individuals are found in the population (Kazazian and Antonarakis 1988, p. 62). The frequency of affected males in the population for quite a few X-linked diseases can be obtained approximately by dividing the length of the coding sequence (in base pairs) by 70 million (e.g., for Duchenne muscular dystrophy, 14,000/70,000,000 = 0.0002, or 1 in 5,000 males).

Computer programs used to calculate risks often request information regarding allele frequencies and mutation rates, but they do not always ask for fitness. Although they can calculate all that they need from the data requested, if we are performing a calculation for a disease for which we do not know the mutation rate, what do we enter to approximate the correct level of fitness or the population frequency of carrier mothers? The following formula gives the relationship between the mutation rate to be entered into the computer and the allele frequency (q), where N is the coefficient of μ that we want the computer to assume (e.g., 18μ).

$$\text{Mutation rate} = 2q/N \tag{2.7}$$

As examples, for Duchenne muscular dystrophy, where we assume that the population frequency of female carriers is 4μ, if we are asked instead for allele frequency and mutation rate, we could enter 0.0002 and 0.9998 as the frequency of mutant and normal alleles and 2(0.0002)/

4 = 0.0001 as the mutation rate. For hemophilia A, if we chose 0.00009 as the allele frequency, we could enter 2(0.00009)/18 = 0.00001 as the mutation rate. The calculated frequency of female carriers should be the same whether we use the population frequency of heterozygotes (2pq) or the relevant multiple of the mutation rate. For example, 4μ = 2pq for Duchenne muscular dystrophy or 18μ = 2pq for hemophilia A (18 * 0.00001 = 0.00018 or 2 * 0.99991 * 0.00009 = 0.00018).

When using computer programs, it is important to understand that there may be hidden links between several numbers that we might be asked to provide. For instance, if the allele frequency entered for Duchenne muscular dystrophy is greater than exactly twice the number that we enter for the mutation rate, we may have inadvertently told the computer that males can reproduce ($f > 0$). Similarly, if the mutation rate is ever specified to be 0 (which may be the default value in the program if a value is not entered), the computer has just been told that *all* females directly ancestral to the affected male are obligate carriers. Did you really mean to specify that when the human species first evolved, the progenitor female was a carrier?

To consider pedigree evidence from previous generations (anterior evidence), we need to know how risk is "transmitted up" pedigrees. In familial cases, if the mother's posterior risk of being a carrier was 0.5, this was halved to obtain the daughter's prior risk because the daughter could have inherited either of her mother's X chromosomes with equal likelihood. From this argument, however, it is not immediately clear what the reverse process should be. If the daughter has a posterior risk of $\frac{2}{3}$, was her mother's risk $\frac{4}{3}$, or $\frac{1}{3}$, or what? The answer is that the risk is halved going up the pedigree as well as coming down the pedigree, but the proof of this is worth going through for two reasons: (*a*) I will use it to show a different approach to the analysis of pedigrees, and (*b*) it is particularly worthwhile to show that the risk can still legitimately be halved going from one female up to her female predecessor when $f > 0$ and the possibility exists that the mutation could have been transmitted through the male lineage instead.

In the slightly different layout shown in Figure 2.7 and Table 2.11, we start with the population risk for the grandmother to be a carrier of Duchenne muscular dystrophy ($f = 0$), which is 4μ. The layout continues by splitting both her carrier and noncarrier columns into two, to consider independently the possibility that her daughter, the affected boy's mother, might be a carrier or a noncarrier. Finally, for each of the four combinations, we consider the conditional probability of having the affected son.

In Table 2.11, the carrier risk for the mother is given by adding the joint risks for all columns where the heading states that she is a carrier

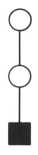

Figure 2.7 A small family in which the grandson has an isolated case of an X-linked recessive, genetically lethal disease. Table 2.11 and the text show that the risk that his grandmother is a carrier is equal to half of the risk that his mother is a carrier.

Table 2.11 Probabilities of combinations of genotypes for the females in Figure 2.7

Grandmother =	Carrier		Noncarrier	
Prior probability	4μ		1	
Mother =	Carrier	Noncarrier	Carrier	Noncarrier
Conditional probability	0.5	0.5	2μ	1
Son affected	0.5	μ	0.5	μ
Joint probability	μ	$2\mu^2$	μ	μ

Note: See the text for the calculation of the posterior risk for each female.

(columns 1 and 3) and dividing by the total for all columns in which she appears (columns 1 to 4, inclusive). The total of columns 1 and 3 is 2μ and the total for all four columns is 3μ (ignoring terms containing μ^2). Her risk is therefore 0.667 (⅔). By a similar process, the grand-mother is a carrier in columns 1 and 2 but not in columns 3 or 4. The total for columns 1 and 2 is μ, which gives her a risk of 0.333 (⅓). It is worthwhile to do the same exercise adding in another generation (starting with his great-grandmother) when there will be eight columns. Each female will be a carrier in a different set of four columns, and the risks should work out to 0.017 (⅙) for the great-grandmother, 0.333 (⅓) for the grandmother, and 0.667 (⅔) for the mother of the isolated, affected male. Remember that new mutations are twice as likely in females (2μ) as in males (μ), (assuming that $\mu = v$), because females have two X chromosomes.

When $f > 0$, as in hemophilia A ($f = 0.7$), we know that the female at the top of the pedigree will have a population carrier risk greater than 4μ (18μ when $f = 0.7$). Using the formulae given above, we can determine that if we are referring to the mother of the affected person, her carrier risk will be 90%. What we want to prove, therefore, is that the grandmother of the affected person has a carrier risk of 45%. In considering this example, we must include an additional column to account for the possibility that the grandfather was affected (Figure 2.8). (Remember, we are considering population risks for people of unknown genotypes. Obviously, if the grandfather in a specific family was known to be healthy, this calculation would not apply. Let us treat the pedigree as if the mother was adopted and we have no information available on the rest of her biological family.)

There are two additional twists to this story: (a) the population probability that an unknown male will have the disease is 10μ (half of his mother's risk of 18μ plus μ for a new mutation in him; also obtained from equation 2.5); and (b) although all daughters of an affected male must be obligate carriers, the probability of his reproducing is only 0.7 when $f = 0.7$ (70% of the time he will have obligate carrier daughters and 30% of the time he will fail to reproduce). This accounts for the figure of 0.7 used for the conditional probability between the affected grandfather and the carrier mother in Table 2.12.

The mother is a carrier in columns 1, 3, and 5 of Table 2.12 and a noncarrier in columns 2, 4, and 6 (columns 2 and 4 can be ignored). Her carrier risk is $9\mu/10\mu$, or 90%. The grandmother is a carrier in columns 1 and 2 only; her risk is therefore $4.5\mu/10\mu$, or 45%. Note that all permutations were considered, however unusual; for example, in column 2, the grandmother was a carrier, the mother was a noncarrier, and the son was affected. This would require two independent mutational events, one leading to the grandmother's being a carrier, the second leading to the son's being affected with an independent mutation.

It is a good general strategy to add a column for every possible combination of genotypes so that none can be missed. At the end, columns containing terms with μ^2 or higher powers are ignored, but following this method, columns that should be counted are not inadvertently omitted. This general procedure will become very important in later sections of the book.

Table 2.13 is similar to Table 2.10 but includes an extra generation. It shows the posterior risk for both grandparents at different values of f (assuming that $\mu = \nu$). The interpretation of Table 2.13 is that if fitness $= 0.7$ and the mother of an isolated case has no knowledge of her family history (e.g., she was adopted), her mother would have been a carrier 45% of the time, her father affected 35% of the time,

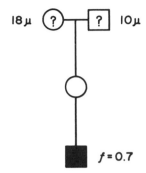

Figure 2.8 A small family in which the grandson has an isolated case of an X-linked recessive disease which is not genetically lethal. In such cases, it is possible that the disease could have been transmitted through the maternal grandfather if his status is not known. Table 2.12 and the text show that the risk that his grandmother is a carrier is still equal to half of the risk that his mother is a carrier.

Table 2.12 Probabilities of combinations of genotypes in Figure 2.8

	Grandmother Carrier		Grandfather Affected		Neither Carrier	
Prior probability	18μ		10μ		1	
Mother =	Carrier	Noncarrier	Carrier	Noncarrier	Carrier	Noncarrier
Conditional probability	0.5	0.5	0.7†	0	2μ	1
Son affected	0.5	μ	0.5	μ	0.5	μ
Joint probability	4.5μ	9μ²	3.5μ	0	μ	μ
Column	1	2	3	4	5	6

†(Probability of reproducing) * (carrier risk if he does) = 0.7 * 1.

and neither parent would have possessed the mutation 20% of the time. The carrier risk for the grandmother is always half of the carrier risk for the mother (see Table 2.10 for posterior risks for the mother). The "carrier" risk for the grandfather obviously applies only if we do not know his clinical status; if we do know his status, his risk is either 0% or 100%.

Now that we have established that we can halve the risk going from one female to the next up a pedigree as well as down a pedigree, we are ready to tackle a situation where the mother of an isolated case has useful anterior information or has relatives who want to know their carrier risks. In Figure 2.9, the consultand, III-5, has a first cousin

Table 2.13   Prior and posterior risks for the grandmother and grandfather of an isolated case at different values for reproductive fitness

	Grandmother Carrier		Grandfather Affected		Neither Carrier
f	Prior	Posterior	Prior	Posterior	Posterior
0	4μ	0.333	3μ†	0.000	0.667
0.1	4.67μ	0.350	3.33μ	0.050	0.600
0.2	5.5μ	0.367	3.75μ	0.100	0.533
0.3	6.57μ	0.383	4.29μ	0.150	0.467
0.4	8μ	0.400	5μ	0.200	0.400
0.5	10μ	0.417	6μ	0.250	0.333
0.6	13μ	0.433	7.5μ	0.300	0.267
0.7	18μ	0.450	10μ	0.350	0.200
0.8	28μ	0.467	15μ	0.400	0.133
0.9	58μ	0.483	30μ	0.450	0.067

†Hypothetical, since he cannot reproduce if affected when $f = 0$.

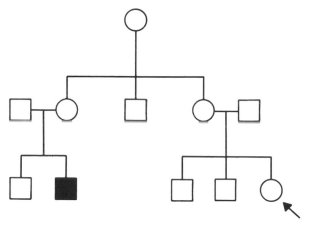

Figure 2.9   A family with an isolated case of an X-linked recessive, genetically lethal disease. Tables 2.14 to 2.21 show several methods of calculating the risk that III-5 is a carrier of the disease. Five different methods (methods A to E) are discussed in the text, all of which give the correct posterior risk for II-4 and III-5 but not necessarily II-2 or I-1.

Table 2.14   Provisional posterior risk for II-2 in Figure 2.9

	Carrier	Noncarrier
Prior probability	4μ	1
Conditional probabilities		
that III-1 is normal	1/2	1
that III-2 is affected	1/2	μ
Joint probability	μ	μ
Posterior probability	1/2	1/2

with a genetically lethal ($f = 0$) X-linked recessive disease and wants to find out her risk of being a carrier of the disease. Since there are many ways to approach the analysis, we will try several different methods to obtain both her risk and the risks for the intervening members of the family and compare their accuracy. There is a shortcut method that people frequently use (method A below). As we shall see, the shortcut works well for assessing distant relatives but not for assessing immediate family members of the affected person. Analysis of good and bad methods is worthwhile at this point, since (*a*) even if you know the answer is wrong, it is often difficult to find where the error has crept in, and (*b*) later chapters contain situations where it may be difficult to find an independent method to check the final answer, and we have to have faith in the logic of the methods applied.

Method A.   Starting with the mother of the affected person, calculate a risk for his grandmother, and then go down to his first cousin, the consultand. We use this modified risk to determine the carrier risk for her mother. The "prior risk" ($\frac{1}{4}$) for I-1 is half of the posterior risk ($\frac{1}{2}$) for her daughter, II-2. We then use this to determine the prior risk of II-4. The prior risk ($\frac{1}{14}$) for II-4 is half of the posterior risk ($\frac{1}{7}$) for her mother, I-1 (Tables 2.14–2.16).

The prior risk for the consultand, III-5, is therefore $\frac{1}{106}$. This is the correct answer for her, and $\frac{1}{53}$ is the correct answer for her mother, but the answers obtained for the posterior risks for females II-2 and I-1 are *not correct*. Because the final answer for III-5 is correct, many students assume that all of the intervening steps must also be correct, which unfortunately is not so.

How can a chain of incorrect answers yield the correct final answer for the consultand? The key is that she and her mother, II-4, are the only people for whom we have used all of the available pedigree information. We used 4μ as the prior risk for II-2, which would be correct

Table 2.15   Provisional posterior risk for I-1 in Figure 2.9

	Carrier	Noncarrier
"Prior risk"	1/4	3/4
Conditional probability that II-3 is normal	1/2	1
Joint probability	1/8	3/4 (= 6/8)
Posterior probability	1/7	6/7

Table 2.16   Calculation of posterior risk for II-4 in Figure 2.9

	Carrier	Noncarrier
Prior probability	1/14	13/14
Conditional probabilities		
that III-3 is normal	1/2	1
that III-4 is normal	1/2	1
Joint probability	1/56	13/14 (= 52/56)
Posterior probability	1/53	52/53

if we had no anterior information for her; however, this is not the case, since her mother has a normal son and a daughter with two normal grandsons. In going from II-2 to II-4, we eventually incorporated all of this information into the calculation, and when this has happened, we get the correct answer. This method is adequate for everyone but the mother of the affected person as long as this limitation is understood. If we decided to make I-1 the consultand instead, we would use II-4 and her two sons as a conditional probability for I-1 ($5/8$; see Table 2.4), since it would now be legal to use that branch of the family at this stage. This would yield the correct answer (taking into account all of the pedigree information) of $5/53$ for I-1, as shown below.

Method B.   To treat the grandmother, I-1, as the consultand, start with the mother of the affected person, move up to the grandmother, and then include posterior information for the grandmother (Table 2.17). We could also have arrived at the same answer by starting with the grandmother instead of the mother of the affected male if we performed a miniature internal Bayesian calculation for the mother of the affected person (see also Tables 2.3 and 2.4).

Table 2.17   Calculation of the posterior risk for I-1 in Figure 2.9, given that the posterior risk for II-2 is 1/2, as calculated in Table 2.14

	Carrier	Noncarrier
Prior probability	1/4	3/4
Conditional probabilities		
II-3	1/2	1
II-4 + sons	5/8	1
Joint probability	5/64	48/64
Posterior probability	5/53	48/53

Table 2.18   Calculation of the posterior risk for I-1 in Figure 2.9

	Carrier	Noncarrier
Prior probability	4μ	1
Conditional probabilities		
II-3	1/2	1
II-4	5/8	1
I-2 + sons	Carrier + Noncarrier	Carrier + Noncarrier
	$(\frac{1}{2} * \frac{1}{2} * \frac{1}{2}) + (\frac{1}{2} * 1 * \mu)$	$(2\mu * \frac{1}{2} * \frac{1}{2}) + (1 * 1 * \mu)$
Joint probability	$5\mu/32$	$3\mu/2 = 48\mu/32$
Posterior probability	5/53	48/53

Method C.   To treat the grandmother, I-1, as the consultand, start with her and consider all of her descendants (including the affected child and his mother) in the conditional probabilities (Table 2.18). Even this additional step does not address the final risk for the mother of the affected male, because we are still treating her prior risk of being a carrier as 4μ, which is correct only when no details of the family history are available. The only way to obtain her correct final risk is to modify her prior risk in a manner that incorporates the known anterior history. To do this, we need to start with her mother, I-1.

Method D.   Starting with the grandmother, use the posterior history to obtain her modified risk and then apply this as the starting point for the mother of the affected person (Table 2.19).

The posterior risk for I-1 is $5\mu/4$. The prior risk for her daughter,

Table 2.19   Calculation of provisional risk for I-1 in Figure 2.9

	Carrier	Noncarrier
Prior probability	4μ	1
Conditional probabilities		
II-2	1/2	1
II-3 + sons	5/8	1
Joint probability	$5\mu/4$	1

Table 2.20   Calculation of posterior risk for II-2 in Figure 2.9

	Carrier	Noncarrier
Prior probability	$2\mu + 5\mu/8$ (new + inherited)	1
Conditional probabilities		
III-1	1/2	1
III-2	1/2	μ
Joint probability	$21\mu/32$	$32\mu/32$
Posterior probability	21/53	32/53

II-2, will therefore be half of this value ($5\mu/8$) plus 2μ. The two components of this risk represent inherited and new mutations in II-2. The probability of II-2 inheriting an existing mutation from her mother is $5\mu/8$ and the probability of a new mutation occurring on either of her two X chromosomes is 2μ (Table 2.20).

Finally, we have found a method that will give the correct posterior risk of $21/53$ for the mother of the affected male. This method, however, is specific to her and cannot be used to derive simultaneously the risks for I-1 or II-4.

A comprehensive method, although admittedly more difficult to write out, is the method of starting at the top of the pedigree and writing out a column for every possible combination of genotypes. We will take the trouble to go through this more complex analysis because it is similar to the method used to calculate probabilities over pedigrees (and then lod scores) and because it represents the foundations of a good strategy to solve some of the more difficult problems posed later. Unlike methods A–D discussed above, this method will also allow us to compute the correct risks for all of the females in the pedigree simultaneously. I recommend this method over all of the others whenever you are not absolutely sure that some of the shorter methods will give the correct answer.

Method E.   Starting with the most senior relevant ancestor, we consider all possible combinations of genotypes separately. To accomplish this, we start at the top of the pedigree and form two columns (carrier and noncarrier) for the "first" female (Table 2.21). Her sons (or in later chapters, biochemical or molecular data pertaining to her) are included under these headings as conditional probabilities. Each time we come to a daughter, we split the column into two (again, carrier and noncarrier, to reflect the uncertainty of their genotypes). Thus for N females in the pedigree, we should have 2^N columns at the end of this process. In the left column, all of the females will be carriers; in the right column, all of the females will be noncarriers; in between, there will be every other permutation, including some that are clearly ridiculous. By considering all possible permutations of genotypes, even the ridiculous, we are assured that we shall overlook none. Furthermore, computers do not understand genetics, so they cannot decide which combinations make sense and which are ridiculous, but they can be programmed quite easily to generate a matrix of all possible permutations of genotypes for a specified family group and to calculate the probability of each of these chains of events, however small. This method, therefore, represents the core of computer analyses, which we discuss in Chapter 6 (gene mapping).

We will ignore the figures in columns 3, 5, 6, 7, 8, 9, 10, 11, 13, 14, and 15, which contain higher powers of μ. This leaves only columns 1, 2, 4, 12, and 16 to consider. I-1 is a carrier in columns 1 to 8 and a noncarrier in columns 9 to 16. Carrier $= \mu/64 + \mu/64 + \mu/8 = 5\mu/32$ and noncarrier $= \mu/2 + \mu = 48\mu/32$. She has a posterior carrier risk of $5/53$ (and a noncarrier risk of $48/53$). II-2 is a carrier in columns 1 to 4 and 9 to 12 and a noncarrier in columns 5 to 8 and 13 to 16. Carrier $= \mu/64 + \mu/64 + \mu/8 + \mu/2 = 21\mu/32$ and noncarrier $= \mu = 32\mu/32$. She has a posterior carrier risk of $21/53$. II-4 is a carrier in columns 1, 2, 5, 6, 9, 10, 13, and 14 and a noncarrier in columns 3, 4, 7, 8, 11, 12, 15, and 16. Carrier $= \mu/64 + \mu/64 = \mu/32$ and noncarrier $= \mu/8 + \mu/2 + \mu = 52\mu/32$. She has a posterior carrier risk of $1/53$. III-5 is a carrier in all odd-numbered columns and a noncarrier in all even-numbered columns. Carrier $= \mu/64$ and noncarrier $= \mu/64 + \mu/8 + \mu/2 + \mu = 105\mu/64$. Her carrier risk is $1/106$.

Using this method, we see that the posterior carrier risk for the mother of the affected male is $21/53$, or 0.396 (39.6%), which is less than the 50% risk apparently assigned by the short-cut method, which

Table 2.21 The probabilities of all combinations of genotypes in Figure 2.9

Row \ Column	1	2	3	4	5	6	7	8	9	10	11	12	13	14	15	16
I-1 =	Carrier								Noncarrier							
Prior risk	4μ								1							
II-3 is normal	$\tfrac{1}{2}$								1							
II-2 =	Carrier				Noncarrier				Carrier				Noncarrier			
Conditional prob.	$\tfrac{1}{2}$				$\tfrac{1}{2}$				2μ				1			
III-1 is normal	$\tfrac{1}{2}$				1				$\tfrac{1}{2}$				1			
III-2 is affected	$\tfrac{1}{2}$				μ				$\tfrac{1}{2}$				μ			
II-4 =	C		NC		C		NC		C		NC		C		NC	
Conditional prob.	2μ		1		2μ		1		2μ		1		2μ		1	
III-3 is normal	$\tfrac{1}{2}$		1		$\tfrac{1}{2}$		1		$\tfrac{1}{2}$		1		$\tfrac{1}{2}$		1	
III-4 is normal	$\tfrac{1}{2}$		1		$\tfrac{1}{2}$		1		$\tfrac{1}{2}$		1		$\tfrac{1}{2}$		1	
III-5 =	C	NC	C	NC	C	NC	C	NC	C	NC	C	NC	C	NC	C	NC
Conditional prob.	$\tfrac{1}{2}$	$\tfrac{1}{2}$	2μ	1	$\tfrac{1}{2}$	$\tfrac{1}{2}$	2μ	1	$\tfrac{1}{2}$	$\tfrac{1}{2}$	2μ	1	$\tfrac{1}{2}$	$\tfrac{1}{2}$	2μ	1
Total	$\mu^2/16$	$\mu^2/16$	$\mu^2/2$	$\mu/4$	$\mu^3/4$	$\mu^3/4$	$2\mu^3$	μ^2	$\mu^2/8$	$\mu^2/8$	μ^2	$\mu/2$	$\mu^2/4$	$\mu^2/4$	$2\mu^2$	μ
Column	1	2	3	4	5	6	7	8	9	10	11	12	13	14	15	16

Note: C = carrier, NC = noncarrier.

ignores her anterior family history. In later chapters, we cover how this type of analysis can be combined with either the results from creatine kinase testing or DNA data or both. When teaching the different validity of these methods, I am often asked "Isn't this method cyclical?" or "Doesn't this method use the daughter to modify her mother's risk and then use this modified risk as a prior risk on the daughter?" The answer is No. The method may appear to do this, but it is an illusion. It actually calculates the probability of all possible genotypic combinations in mother and daughter simultaneously and then obtains the cumulative carrier risk for each person by obtaining the sum of all columns in which that person was assigned a carrier genotype. The result at the foot of one column is not dependent upon what happened in other columns, so no cycling is involved.

3

Incorporation of Females with Biochemical Test Results into Bayesian Calculations

In this chapter we consider the combination of biochemical test results (or results of other tests that depend upon the phenotype) with Bayesian probability, which depends upon the reproductive history and is therefore an indirect indicator of the probable genotype.

3.1 Linearity of the Test Results

It is necessary to know whether the test results follow a linear scale or a Gaussian or similar distribution. If the results are expressed as a percentage risk, they are linear. A female with a biochemical test result that gives her a 60% risk of being a carrier has precisely double the likelihood of being a carrier of a female with a 30% risk. However, a female with a creatine kinase (CK) level of 60 does not necessarily have double the risk of a female with a level of 30. The crude units (CK level, F8C activity, etc.) do not relate to risk in a linear fashion. It is much easier to include biochemical test results in Bayesian calculations if the results are part of a linear scale. Gaussian distributions can be converted to linear functions by a logistic equation.

$$\log [P/(1 - P)] = \text{Constant} * (\text{Gaussian test result}) + \text{constant}$$

P is the probability of being a carrier, and the constants are determined empirically by studying appropriately sized collections of obli-

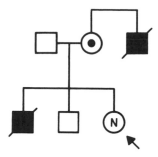

Figure 3.1   A family with Duchenne muscular dystrophy. The daughter, II-3, has a "normal" level of creatine kinase. The calculation of the risk that the daughter is a carrier is shown in Table 3.1.

Table 3.1   Calculation of carrier risk for II-3 in Figure 3.1

	Carrier	Noncarrier
Prior probability	0.5	0.5
Conditional probability		
normal CK†	0.333	0.95
Joint probability	0.167	0.475
Posterior probability	0.26	0.74

Note: Noncarrier: carrier ratio = 2.85.
†CK = creatine kinase.

gate carriers and normal females. Simple separation into carrier and noncarrier categories (such as declaring females above or below a specific threshold to be carriers or noncarriers) is clearly nonlinear and should be avoided if at all possible. If this is not possible, the numbers placed in the columns should represent the non-false-positive and the false-negative situations. For example, if 1 out of 3 carriers of Duchenne muscular dystrophy has a "normal" level of CK and 1 out of 20 noncarriers has an "abnormal" level, the conditional probability for a female to have a normal CK result is 0.333 ($\frac{1}{3}$) in her carrier column (false-negative) result and 0.95 ($\frac{19}{20}$) in her noncarrier column (non-false-positive result, i.e., true negative) (Figure 3.1 and Table 3.1). These numbers can be normalized to 0.26 carrier and 0.74 noncarrier or a ratio of 1 to 2.85, or 0.3514.

  A normal CK test result, using these particular values for error rates, reduces a female's risk of being a carrier of Duchenne muscular dystrophy slightly more than if she had one unaffected son (ratio 2.0; posterior risks 0.33 to 0.67). As already stated, a continuous scale of risks would be much more desirable than arbitrary cutoff values of $\frac{1}{3}$ and $\frac{19}{20}$ (or whatever other values a laboratory happens to choose for its cutoff; these happen to be the numbers normally quoted for potential carriers of Duchenne muscular dystrophy to fall outside 2 standard deviations from the norm for CK M activity).

3.2 Column Ratios

The noncarrier/carrier ratio between the columns for a normal male in a Bayesian calculation is 2.0 (0.5 in the carrier column and 1.0 in the noncarrier column); the same ratio for an affected male would be extremely low (0.5 in the carrier column and μ in the noncarrier column). If μ has a numerical value of 10^{-6}, the ratio is 0.000002. The ratios defined by unaffected and affected males are therefore far from being symmetrical. As stated in the section on new mutations, this very low ratio is countered by the very low population frequency of carriers.

It is assumed that the phenotypes of males in almost all X-linked conditions are absolutely indicative of their genotypes. This is not so for females unless there is proof that they are obligate carriers. The column ratio for a female who is being used as a conditional probability in a Bayesian calculation, therefore, should not exceed the maximum ratio determined by males. A female with a carrier risk of 10% should not have 0.1 placed in her mother's carrier column and 0.9 placed in the noncarrier column; this would be a noncarrier to carrier ratio of 9, equivalent in weighting to more than three unaffected brothers, who would have a total ratio of 8 (2 * 2 * 2). Instead, she should exert a ratio slightly less than 2.0 (actually 1.8, or 90% of 2) (Table 3.2). It does not matter whether the numbers entered are 1 and 1.8 or 1000 and 1800 or the normalized values of 0.357 and 0.643 as long as the ratio between them is 1.8 and the lower number goes in the carrier column.

If she had a carrier risk of 90% instead, the lower number (0.167, obtained by reversing the conditional probabilities in Table 3.2) would be placed in the noncarrier column (and 0.833 in the carrier column), so the overall trend favors carrier status in her mother (section 3.5 explains why the ratio 90% carrier to 10% noncarrier "counts more" than 10% carrier to 90% noncarrier). The ratio applied to the mother when a daughter has a normal CK level should be 1.48 (74% of 2.0; see above for the derivation of the 74%; this can also be demonstrated by inserting conditional probabilities of $\frac{1}{3}$ and $\frac{19}{20}$ instead of 0.1 and 0.9 in the calculation above). This represents the maximum ratio set

Table 3.2   Influence of a daughter's biochemical test result on her mother's risk of being a carrier

	Mother			
	Carrier		Noncarrier	
Prior risk	0.5		0.5	
Daughter =	Carrier	Noncarrier	Carrier	Noncarrier
Prior probability	0.5	0.5	2μ	1
Conditional probability biochemical test	0.1	0.9	0.1	0.9
Joint probability	0.025	0.225	≈ 0	0.45

Notes: Mother's carrier total = 0.25 (posterior risk = 0.357); mother's noncarrier total = 0.45 (posterior risk = 0.643); noncarrier·carrier ratio = 0.45/0.25 = 1.8

by what a normal son would count reduced to reflect the degree of uncertainty surrounding how well the daughter's phenotype indicates her true genotype. It follows from the above argument that females with a carrier risk of 50% should not exert any overall influence on their mother's carrier risk (they should have a ratio of 1.0).

3.3   Biochemical Tests on the Consultand Herself

Results of tests on the female who is the subject of the Bayesian calculation can be entered directly without the above restrictions, and the magnitude of the column ratio is limited only by the discriminatory powers of the test. As an example, an abnormal CK result increases the likelihood that a female is a carrier by a factor of 13.3 to 1 (Table 3.3).

3.4   Stating Conditional Probabilities in Words

As in all other aspects of Bayesian calculations, there is less chance of entering the wrong numbers if the assumption of the conditional probability can be clearly stated in words. All of the following conditional probabilities apply to a mother at 50% prior risk. The condition stated for each of the following situations assumes that the following words are implied before and after each statement "The probability

Table 3.3   The effect of biochemical test results on the consultand

	Carrier	Noncarrier
Prior probability	1/2	1/2
Conditional probability		
normal CK† result	2/3	1/20
Joint probability	1/3 = 40/120	1/40 = 3/120
Posterior probability	40/43	3/43

Note: Noncarrier/carrier ratio = 3/40 = 0.075.
†CK = creatine kinase.

Table 3.4   Conditional probabilities for various events if the mother is a carrier or a noncarrier

	Mother		Noncarrier:
The probability that	Carrier	Noncarrier	Carrier Ratio
a son is normal	0.5	1.0	2.0000
a daughter has a 10% risk of being a			
carrier based upon some test	0.357	0.643	1.8000
a daughter has a 90% risk of being			
carrier based upon some test	0.833	0.167	0.2000
a son is affected	0.5	µ	Low†
a daughter is an obligate carrier	0.5	2µ	Low†
the mother herself will have normal CK‡	0.26	0.74	2.8500
a daughter will have normal CK	0.403	0.597	1.4805
the mother will have abnormal CK	0.93	0.07	0.0750
a daughter will have abnormal CK	0.878	0.122	0.1395

†These conditions would make the mother an obligate carrier.
‡CK = creatine kinase.

that . . . ," ". . . if the mother is a carrier or if the mother is a noncarrier" (Table 3.4).

3.5   Resolution of Conflicting Evidence

When there is conflicting evidence pertaining to carrier status, as a general rule, the evidence favoring carrier status counts more strongly. I say this based upon mathematical reality rather than the urge to be

Table 3.5 Effect upon their mother of two daughters, one with a normal test result and one with an abnormal test result

| | Mother | | Noncarrier: Carrier Ratio |
	Carrier	Noncarrier	
Prior probability	0.5	0.5	1.0
Conditional probabilities			
daughter with abnormal result	0.878	0.122	0.139
daughter with normal result	0.403	0.597	1.481
Joint probability	0.176917	0.036417	0.206
Posterior probability	0.829	0.171	0.206

overly cautious when advising women that they are unlikely to be carriers. As an obvious example, if a mother at 50% risk of being a carrier of hemophilia B has two sons, one affected, the other not, the normal son reduces the mother's carrier risk by a factor of 2.0, but the affected son raises her risk by such an enormous ratio $(0.5 : \mu)$ that we assume that she is an obligate carrier of the disease. If we assume that the mutation rate is 1 in 200,000, the affected son has a weighting 50,000 times greater in this calculation than his normal brother. As a second example (Table 3.5), if a mother at 50% risk of being a carrier of Duchenne muscular dystrophy has two daughters, one with a normal CK result, the other an abnormal one, the first daughter exerts an noncarrier:carrier ratio of 1.48; the second daughter exerts a ratio of 0.139. Their combined influence is 0.206, or almost 5 to 1 in favor of the mother's being a carrier.

Since the ratio is always in the form of $1:R$ for C:NC, normalized posterior risks can be obtained from the final ratio (R) by the formulae

Carrier $= 1/(1 + R)$
Noncarrier $= R/(1 + R)$.

It was stressed earlier that the ratio between the columns is critical, whereas the absolute values of conditional risks are irrelevant to the outcome of a Bayesian calculation. It does not matter whether a normal male has the number 0.5 or 5,000 or 0.0001 entered into the carrier column when he is used as a conditional probability for his mother as long as the number entered under her noncarrier column is twice as big. The ratio matters; it must always be 2 (noncarrier:carrier). When we are considering DNA-based evidence in the next few chapters or calculating lod scores or probabilities over pedigrees under gene-mapping methodology, the absolute values of the numbers are often very, very small, but the ratio of 10^{-15} to $2 * 10^{-15}$ is the same as the ratio of 0.5 to 1.0.

3.6 Noncarrier Ratios

If you are wondering why I have written everything as a noncarrier ratio instead of a carrier ratio, Figure 3.2 and Table 3.6 will illustrate the reason.

The little trick performed as we changed generations where the new ratio is twice the old ratio plus 1 was first noticed empirically, but it can be demonstrated algebraically as follows: let $R1 = NC/C$ and let $R2 = NC'/C'$ where $R1$ is the noncarrier ratio for the previous generation and $R2$ is the noncarrier ratio for the new generation. The prior carrier risk for the new generation is half of the posterior risk for the old ($C' = C/2$), and the prior noncarrier risk is the old noncarrier risk plus the second half of the old carrier risk ($NC' = NC + C/2$). Therefore, $R2 = NC'/C' = [NC + C/2]/[C/2] = [2(NC) + C]/C = 2(NC/C) + C/C = 2(R1) + 1$. A similar method could be derived for the carrier ratio instead of the noncarrier ratio, but it is much more complicated because the denominator is complex ($2NC + C$ instead of C). The main advantage to doing the noncarrier ratios in parallel to the Bayesian calculation is that it is a *simple* check. For instance, if (like me) you have an inborn tendency to halve the joint risk instead of halving the normalized posterior risk when changing generations, you will be alerted to the error when the Bayesian answer does not agree with the answer obtained by the ratio method. For practice, you could try this method on the pedigree in Figure 2.3. Carrier ratios work just as well as noncarrier ratios as long as no change in generations is required.

In Figure 3.3, two females are interested in their risk of being a carrier of Duchenne muscular dystrophy. Both have had several CK tests performed with results in the normal range. The laboratory performing the tests quotes its false-negative and false-positive rates as $1/3$ and $1/20$, the latter being the fraction of noncarriers above 2 standard deviations from their norm. I-2 is an obligate carrier. II-2 is the daughter of an obligate carrier who has the following conditional factors in her favor: normal CK, two normal sons, a daughter with normal CK, and a normal grandson (Table 3.7). III-3 is the granddaughter of an obligate carrier. Her prior risk is half of her mother's posterior risk (omitting the daughter's branch of the family from that calculation) modified by the facts that she has normal CK and a normal son (Table 3.8).

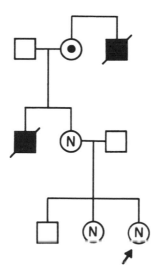

Figure 3.2   A family with Duchenne muscular dystrophy. Females II-2, III-2, and III-3 all have "normal" levels of creatine kinase (CK). The risk that III-3 is a carrier is calculated in Table 3.6. This calculation takes into account three types of evidence: (a) her mother has normal CK, (b) her mother has a healthy son and a daughter with normal CK, and (c) the consultand herself has normal CK.

Table 3.6   Calculation of the posterior risk for III-3 in Figure 3.2, based upon the posterior risk for her mother, II-2

II 2 =	Carrier	Noncarrier	Noncarrier: Carrier Ratio
Prior probability	0.5	0.5	1.0
Conditional probabilities			
son III-1	0.5	1.0	2.0
normal CK†	0.26	0.74	2.85
daughter III-2	0.403	0.597	1.48
Joint probability	0.026195	0.22089	8.436
Posterior probability	0.106	0.894	8.436

III-3 =	Carrier	Noncarrier	
Prior probability	0.053	0.947	2(8.436) + 1 = 17.872
Conditional probability			
normal CK	0.26	0.74	2.85
Joint probability	0.01378	0.70078	50.9352
Posterior probability	0.0193 (1.93%)	0.9807	50.9352

†CK = creatine kinase.

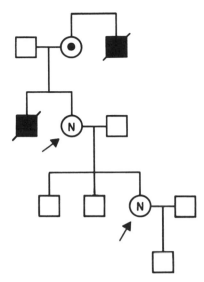

Figure 3.3 A family with Duchenne muscular dystrophy. Reproductive history and biochemical test results are combined in Tables 3.7 and 3.8 to calculate the risks that II-2 and III-3 are carriers.

Table 3.7 Calculation of the posterior risk for II-2 in Figure 3.3

II-2 =	Carrier	Noncarrier	Noncarrier: Carrier Ratio
Prior probability	1/2	1/2	1.00
Conditional probabilities			
CK† result for II-2	1/3	19/20	2.85
son III-1	1/2	1	2.00
son III-2	1/2	1	2.00
III-3 (CK + IV-1)	$(1/2 * 1/2 * 1/3) +$ $(1/2 * 1 * 19/20) = 67/120$	$1 * 1 * 19/20$ $= 114/120$	1.70
Joint probability	$67/2880 = 0.0232638$	$2166/4800 = 0.45125$	19.39
Posterior probability	0.0490266 (4.9%)	0.9509733	19.39

†CK = creatine kinase.

Table 3.8   Calculation of the provisional risk for II-2 and the posterior risk for III-3 in Figure 3.3

II-2 =	Carrier	Noncarrier	Noncarrier: Carrier Ratio
Prior probability	1/2	1/2	1.00
Conditional probability			
CK† result for II-2	1/3	19/20	2.85
son III-1	1/2	1	2.00
son III-2	1/2	1	2.00
Joint probability	1/24 = 5/120	19/40 = 57/120	11.40
Posterior probability	5/62	57/62	11.40

III-3 =	Carrier	Noncarrier	
Prior probability	5/124	119/124	2(11.40) + 1 = 23.80
Conditional probability			
CK result for III 3	1/3	19/20	2.85
son IV-1	1/2	1	2.00
Joint probability	5/744	2261/2480	135.66
	50/7440	6783/7440	
Posterior probability	50/6833	6783/6833	135.66
	0.007317	0.992683	
	(0.73%)		

†CK = creatine kinase.

As before, the conditional risk for III-3 under her mother's carrier column represents a "mini-Bayesian," which is the sum of the independent probabilities (prior * normal son * "normal" CK) if she is a carrier ($\frac{1}{2} * \frac{1}{2} * \frac{1}{3}$) or if she is a noncarrier ($\frac{1}{2} * 1 * \frac{19}{20}$) = $\frac{1}{12}$ + $\frac{19}{40}$ = $\frac{67}{120}$.

3.7   Negative Family History

In situations where there is a negative family history, any type of biochemical or other descriptive test becomes an extremely valuable addition to the basic pedigree risks. Figure 3.4 is the same pedigree that we examined in Figure 2.9. Let us assume this time, however, that the affected male has adrenoleukodystrophy (ALD) and that III-5 is adamant that she does not want to risk having children if she is a carrier. Childhood ALD is a genetic lethal, but within the same kindred there can also be an adult-onset form (caused by the same mutation),

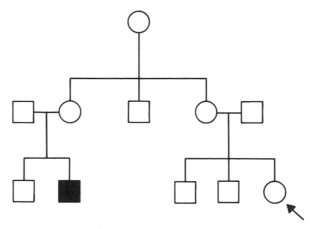

Figure 3.4   A family with an isolated case of adrenoleukodystrophy and/or adrenomyeloneuropathy. The risks for all of the females are calculated in Tables 3.9
(reproductive history only, assuming that the combined reproductive fitness for
both types of the disease is 0.4) and 3.10 (reproductive history plus biochemical
test results, assuming a false-negative rate of 0.2 in females only).

called adrenomyeloneuropathy (AMN), in which males can reproduce.
Let us assume that $f = 0.4$ for all males who possess the mutation.
There is a biochemical test available (increased levels of very long
chain fatty acids, VLCFAs, in plasma and in various tissues) that we
will assume detects all males carrying the mutation and 80% of females. There are no false positives.

Before proceeding with any laboratory tests, we determine the pedigree risk for III-5. This has been written out in the probability of
pedigree format (Table 3.9) so that the biochemical test results can be
inserted later as extra lines, where appropriate. If $f = 0.4$, equation
2.4 or Table 2.10 gives a population risk of 8μ for I-1.

As in section 2.4, we will ignore any column containing terms with
μ^2 or μ^3, which leaves only columns 1 ($\frac{1}{32}$), 2 ($\frac{1}{32}$), 4 ($\frac{8}{32}$), 12 ($\frac{16}{32}$),
and 16 ($\frac{32}{32}$) to consider (total $= \frac{58}{32}$). I-1 is a carrier in columns 1, 2,
and 4 (risk $= \frac{10}{58} = 0.1724$); II-2 is a carrier in columns 1, 2, 4, and
12 (risk $= \frac{26}{58} = 0.4483$); II-4 is a carrier in columns 1 and 2 only (risk
$= \frac{2}{58} = 0.03448$); and III-5 is a carrier in column 1 only (risk $= \frac{1}{58}$
$= 0.01724$).

Although the pedigree risk for III-5 is fairly low (1.7%), the family
elects to proceed with biochemical testing, and let us assume that
females I-1, II-2, II-4, and III-5 have all been tested biochemically
with negative results. Furthermore, since the disease is not evident
from birth and may have adult onset, we also need to establish the
carrier status of all the relevant males as well. Let us assume that II-3,

Table 3.9 Calculation of pedigree probabilities for Figure 3.4 (without results from biochemical tests)

	1	2	3	4	5	6	7	8	9	10	11	12	13	14	15	16
I-1 =	Carrier								Noncarrier							
II-2 =	Carrier				Noncarrier				Carrier				Noncarrier			
II-4 =	C		NC		C		NC		C		NC		C		NC	
III-5 =	C	NC	C	NC	C	NC	C	NC	C	NC	C	NC	C	NC	C	NC
Prior risk	8μ								1							
II-3 normal	½								1							
Conditional prob.	½				½				2μ				1			
III-1 normal	½				1				½				1			
III-2 affected	½				μ				½				μ			
Conditional prob.	½		½		½		½		2μ		1		2μ		1	
III-3 normal	½		1		½		1		½		1		½		1	
III-4 normal	½		1		½		1		½		1		½		1	
Conditional prob.	½	½	2μ	1	½	½	2μ	1	½	½	2μ	1	½	½	2μ	1
Total	μ/32	μ/32	μ²/2	μ/4	μ²/8	μ²/8	2μ³	μ²	μ²/8	μ²/8	μ²	μ/2	μ²/4	μ²/4	2μ²	μ
Column	1	2	3	4	5	6	7	8	9	10	11	12	13	14	15	16

Note: C = carrier, NC = noncarrier.

Table 3.10 Calculation of probabilities for Figure 3.4 including biochemical test results

I-1 =	Carrier	Noncarrier
Prior risk	8μ	1
Conditional prob.		
Biochemical	0.2	1
II-3 normal	½	1

II-2 =	Carrier	Noncarrier	Carrier	Noncarrier
Conditional prob.	½	½	2μ	1
Biochemical	0.2	1	0.2	1
III-1 normal	½	1	½	1
III-2 affected	½	μ	½	μ

II-4 =	C	NC	C	NC	C	NC	C	NC
Conditional prob.	½	2μ	½	2μ	2μ	1	2μ	1
Biochemical	0.2	1	0.2	1	0.2	1	0.2	1
III-3 normal	½	1	½	1	½	1	½	1
III-4 normal	½	1	½	1	½	1	½	1

III-5 =	C	NC	C	NC	C	NC	C	NC	C	NC	C	NC	C	NC	C	NC
Conditional prob.	½	½	½	½	½	½	½	½	½	½	½	½	½	½	½	½
Biochemical	0.2	1	0.2	1	0.2	1	0.2	1	0.2	1	0.2	1	0.2	1	0.2	1
Total†	$\mu/2E4$	$\mu/4E3$	$\mu^2/250$	$\mu/E2$	$\mu^2/E3$	$\mu^2/2E2$	$2\mu^3/25$	$\mu^2/5$	$\mu^2/E3$	$\mu^2/2E2$	$\mu^2/25$	$\mu/10$	$\mu^2/E2$	$\mu^2/20$	$2\mu^2/5$	$\mu/16$
Column	1	2	3	4	5	6	7	8	9	10	11	12	13	14	15	16

Note: C = carrier, NC = noncarrier.
†Exponential nomenclature is used: $E3 = 10^3$, $2E5 = 2 * 10^5$, or 200,000, etc.

III-1, III-3, III-4, and (although he is not on the diagram) the grand-father were all tested and found to have normal levels of VLCFAs (100% accurate in males). We can add lines under the conditional risk for each female to represent the results of her biochemical test (Table 3.10).

As before, we will ignore any column containing terms with μ^2 or μ^3, which leaves only columns 1 (1/20,000), 2 (5/20,000), 4 (200/20,000), 12 (2000/20,000), and 16 (20,000/20,000) to consider (total = 22,206/20,000). I-1 is a carrier in columns 1, 2, and 4 (risk = 206/22,206 = 0.009277); II-2 is a carrier in columns 1, 2, 4, and 12 (risk = 2,206/22,206 = 0.09934); II-4 is a carrier in columns 1 and 2 only (risk = 6/22,206 = 0.0002702); and III-5 is a carrier in column 1 only (risk = 1/22,206 = 0.00004503). The risk that III-5 is a carrier is therefore 0.0045%. Note that unlike the risks based upon pedigree analysis only, her risk is less than half of her mother's risk because she now has conditional data that apply directly to her.

Although no DNA testing was described here, it should be made clear that this case, like the cases studied with Duchenne muscular dystrophy, is given for the sake of example only: extremely accurate DNA testing is available for both diseases.

4

Pedigree Risks

in Autosomal Conditions

4.1 Autosomal Dominant Inheritance

Autosomal dominant conditions are defined as those in which heterozygotes manifest symptoms or characteristics of the condition. From the point of view of calculating genetic risk, the important point is simply that the disease-causing allele need be inherited from only one (affected) parent. The offspring of an affected parent therefore have a 50% chance of inheriting the mutant allele (the genotype) from that parent. The risk of developing symptoms (the phenotype), however, is not necessarily so straightforward. It is necessary to define some terms used in describing the possible effects of an autosomal dominant mutation upon a person; in all cases, we are referring to a heterozygote who does possess the mutation.

Penetrance is used to describe whether a person shows symptoms or not (all or nothing). If the disease does not show full penetrance, it is possible to possess a mutant genotype but never develop the mutant phenotype (e.g., nonpenetrant carriers of polydactyly do not suddenly grow a sixth finger during childhood or in adult life). The most obvious pedigree-based evidence for nonpenetrance is a normal individual with an affected parent and an affected child. A disease may be described as showing 70% penetrance, which means that 70% of heterozygotes will have symptoms and 30% will not (these are obviously population-based statistics, individuals must be either penetrant or nonpenetrant).

Expressivity is used to describe the different degree to which different people are affected. As an example, people with neurofibromatosis (NF-1) may have almost no symptoms (e.g., multiple café au lait spots and no or very few neurofibromas) or they may have very severe symptoms (e.g., up to a few thousand neurofibromas, some of which might cause major disfigurement and disability). To have any level of expression of the disorder, you must be penetrant. Variable expressivity is frequently described in the form of tables indicating the percentage of individuals who have each of the variable diagnostic symptoms (e.g., 28% of individuals with Treacher Collins syndrome have conductive deafness, 32% have cleft palate, and 5% have mental retardation [Connor and Ferguson-Smith 1987, p. 154]).

If the disease is of the type whose symptoms do not develop until later in life, it is possible that a heterozygote who eventually will become affected is not yet old enough to display symptoms. *Age at onset* is a characteristic that applies to such diseases. As an example, Huntington disease is an autosomal dominant disease with 100% penetrance ($P = 1.0$) but a variable age at onset (A-O). All people who inherit the mutant allele will exhibit the mutant phenotype if given sufficient time: some heterozygotes might have symptoms at age 30, more will have them at age 40, more still at age 50, and virtually all are symptomatic by age 70. Age at onset and penetrance are genetically different concepts that in the literature are frequently considered to be interchangeable (age at onset is often treated as the equivalent of penetrance that increases with age); this is not so, although there are many situations where risk calculations proceed along the same lines. It must be emphasized, however, that the genetic counseling differs considerably; as we shall see in the next few calculations, a numerically identical risk of 15% has a very different interpretation depending upon which mechanism applies. Finally, there are some autosomal dominant conditions where penetrance is not complete and for which there is also a variable age at onset.

The situation might arise where one or more affected children are born to two apparently healthy parents. There are several potential explanations to consider for such a phenomenon, the likelihood of which will depend upon what is known about the penetrance, age at onset, mutation rate, etc., for that disease. If there is only one affected child, a new mutation is a much more probable explanation than it is if there are more affected children. If there is more than one affected child, germline mosaicism or nonpenetrance in a parent is a more likely explanation. Germline mosaicism is equally likely in families with just one affected child, of course, but then there is no pedigree-based evidence to substantiate its presence.

Figure 4.1 shows two apparently healthy children who are the offspring of an affected mother. If penetrance is complete, there is nothing further to consider: clearly they have not inherited the mutation

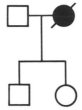

Figure 4.1   A family with an autosomal dominant disease which may exhibit either nonpenetrance or delayed onset. The risk that II-1 is a heterozygote is calculated for either mechanism in Table 4.1.

Table 4.1   Calculation of the posterior risk that an asymptomatic male (II-1) is heterozygous for an autosomal dominant disorder

	Heterozygous	Normal
Mechanism = Nonpenetrance		
Prior probability	0.5	0.5
Conditional probability		
that he is normal	0.2	1.0
Joint probability	0.1	0.5
Posterior probability	0.167	0.833
Mechanism = Delayed Onset		
Prior probability	0.5	0.5
Conditional probability		
that he is still normal	0.2	1.0
Joint probability	0.1	0.5
Posterior probability	0.167	0.833

from her. If penetrance is not complete or if the disease might have delayed onset, there are two possibilities to consider for each child: (*a*) either the child has a normal genotype or (*b*) the child has a mutant genotype but currently a normal phenotype due to nonpenetrance (will never develop symptoms) or because he or she is below the age at which symptoms will manifest themselves (but will eventually develop symptoms). In Table 4.1 we consider each of these scenarios for the first child, assuming either that $P = 0.8$ or that he has attained an age at which 80% of heterozygotes are affected.

Both mechanisms give the same posterior risk of having a mutant genotype; however, this is deceptive. In the former case, where we considered nonpenetrance, he will not subsequently develop symptoms, and the calculation is really relevant only to other members of his family (in particular his future children). In the latter case, where

Table 4.2 Calculation of the risk that an asymptomatic male is a nonpenetrant heterozygote for a congenital disease or that he will still develop symptoms for an adult-onset disease

	Heterozygous		Normal
Prior probability		0.5	0.5
	Affected/ Penetrant	Presymptomatic/ Nonpenetrant	
Conditional probability	0.8	0.2	1.0
Joint probability	0.4	0.1	0.5
Posterior probability	Ignore	0.167	0.833

we considered delayed onset, the fact that he has not developed symptoms yet does not preclude his doing so in the future. Actually there is an interesting paradox in such calculations: although we have used conditional information to reduce his probability of being a heterozygote, the lower his risk, the sooner he will develop symptoms if in fact he actually is one of the remaining heterozygotes who are still presymptomatic. If we perform the calculation in a slightly different manner (Table 4.2), the difference between the two mechanisms can be emphasized.

Since he has a normal phenotype, the column that would require him to have an abnormal phenotype is ignored. If nonpenetrance is the mechanism, the probability that he is a nonpenetrant heterozygote is NP/(NP + NOR), or 0.1/0.6 = 0.167. If delayed onset is the mechanism, the probability that he is a presymptomatic heterozygote is PRE/ (PRE + NOR), or 0.1/0.6 = 0.167. In the latter case, however, this is the risk that he personally will still develop symptoms (and as noted above, if he is going to, he will not have long to wait).

In the above calculations, the conditional probability was always the probability of being normal, which is $1 - P$; P is the probability of being affected. The probability that the child of an affected individual will have a mutant genotype is 0.5, the probability that the child will be affected is $0.5(P)$, and the probability that the child will be a nonpenetrant heterozygote is $0.5(1 - P)$. Since the probability that a child will be homozygous normal is 0.5, the combined probability of being without symptoms is $0.5 + 0.5(1 - P)$. This last formula will be used in the next calculation.

In Figure 4.2, there are two potential calculations: one for II-1, the other for his daughter. Let us start with II-1, for whom there are two different types of conditional probability: the probability that he is

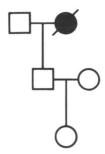

Figure 4.2 A family with an autosomal dominant disease that has a penetrance of 60%. The probabilities that II-1 and III-1 are nonpenetrant heterozygotes are calculated in Tables 4.3 and 4.4. Table 4.4 also shows the calculation of the risk that III-1 would be affected by the disease, had this been a prenatal test instead.

Table 4.3   Calculation of the risk for II-1 in Figure 4.2

	Heterozygous	Normal
Prior probability	0.5	0.5
Conditional probabilities		
that II-1 is normal	0.4	1.0
that III-1 is normal	0.5 + 0.5(0.4)	1.0
Joint probability	0.14	0.5
Posterior probability	0.219	0.781

normal and the probability that his daughter, III-1, is normal (Table 4.3). Assume that $P = 0.6$.

If instead we were to perform the calculation for III-1, we would first obtain a posterior risk for her father and then multiply that by 0.5 and by P to obtain the risk that she will be affected (if this was a prenatal analysis) or by 0.5 and $1 - P$ to obtain the risk that she is a nonpenetrant heterozygote (for reproductive decisions by an apparently healthy person) (Table 4.4).

When there are other people to consider in generation III, the same guidelines are followed as with X-linked diseases (section 2.3): all branches of the family except the one containing the consultand should be used to determine the posterior risk for the consultand's parent. Following this step, conditional information about the consultand may then be incorporated.

In Figure 4.3, we have added a second person in generation III. The calculation of the probability that II-1 is a nonpenetrant heterozygote

Table 4.4   Calculation of the risk for III-1 in Figure 4.2

	Heterozygous			Normal
	Calculation for II-1			
Prior probability	0.5			0.5
Conditional probability				
that II-1 is normal	0.4			1.0
Joint probability	0.2			0.5
Posterior probability	0.2857			0.7143
	Calculation for III-1			
	II-1 heterozygous			II-1 homozygous
Conditional probability	0.2857			0.7143
	Heterozygous		Normal	
Conditional probability	0.5		0.5	1.0
	Affected	Nonpenetrant		
Conditional probability	0.6	0.4	1.0	1.0
Joint probability	0.0857	0.0571	0.1429	0.7143

Notes: Posterior (prenatal) = 8.6% of being affected, 14.2% heterozygous; posterior (postnatal) = 0.0571/0.9143 = 0.0624 = 6.2% risk of being a nonpenetrant heterozygote.

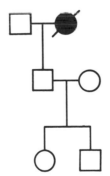

Figure 4.3   A family with an autosomal dominant disease that has a penetrance of 60%. The probabilities that II-1 and III-2 are nonpenetrant heterozygotes are calculated in Tables 4.5 and 4.6.

Table 4.5   Calculation of the risk that II-1 in Figure 4.3 is
heterozygous (calculation for II-1 only)

	Heterozygous	Normal
Prior probability	0.5	0.5
Conditional probability		
that II-1 is normal	0.4	1.0
that III-1 is normal	0.5 + 0.5(0.4)	1.0
that III-2 is normal	0.5 + 0.5(0.4)	1.0
Joint probability	0.098	0.5
Posterior probability	0.164	0.836

is essentially the same as that given above, with the addition of another line under conditional risks to represent his second child, III-2 (Table 4.5). If we were to calculate the risk that III 2 will be affected (prenatal) or is a nonpenetrant heterozygote (postnatal), we can only use III-1 as a conditional probability for II-1 (Table 4.6).

In Figure 4.4, the parents are not affected. There are several possible reasons for this, including nonpaternity, new mutation, germline mosaicism (which is a specific subcategory of new mutation), and nonpenetrance. If penetrance is known to be complete for this disorder, nonpenetrance is ruled out, and either there has been a new mutation (meiotic or mitotic) or there is some non-Mendelian explanation, such as nonpaternity. Under such circumstances, we could attempt to identify the disease-causing mutation if the gene has been cloned and sequenced or to show that subsequent offspring have inherited both opposite parental haplotypes (1 in 4 chance) if there are linked markers. Failing this, we must resort to empirical recurrence risks, which will fall somewhere on the extremely wide spectrum between 2μ and 0.5. (Technically, clinical testing is ruled out when penetrance genuinely equals 1.0, since that should be an all-or-nothing situation; anything in between would be variable expressivity not nonpenetrance. However, diseases do not necessarily fall into such rigid theoretical criteria, and clinical tests might be of considerable value.)

If nonpenetrance has been a reported phenomenon for this disease, the situation becomes even more complex unless some direct test of genotype is available. With the potential of nonpenetrance, a parent could be an asymptomatic heterozygote for the disease. There are several different formulae for calculating recurrence risks, which differ mostly in their treatment of the genetic fitness of penetrant and/or

Table 4.6 Calculation of the risk that III-2 in Figure 4.3 is heterozygous including the probability of being affected

	Heterozygous			Normal
	Calculation for II-1			
Prior probability	0.5			0.5
Conditional probability				
that II-1 is normal	0.4			1.0
that III-1 is normal	0.5 + 0.5(0.4)			1.0
Joint probability	0.14			0.5
Posterior probability	0.219			0.781
	Calculation for III-2			
	II-1 heterozygous			II-1 homozygous
Conditional probability	0.219			0.781
	Heterozygous		Normal	
Conditional probability	0.5		0.5	1.0
	Affected	Nonpenetrant		
Conditional probability	0.6	0.4	1.0	1.0
Joint probability	0.0657	0.0438	0.1095	0.781

Notes: Posterior (prenatal) = 6.6% affected, 11% heterozygous; posterior (postnatal) = 0.0438/0.9343 = 0.0469 = 4.7% risk of being a nonpenetrant heterozygote.

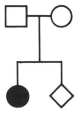

Figure 4.4 A family with an isolated case of an autosomal dominant disease. Possible explanations for the structure of this family along with the risk of recurrence in the fetus are discussed in the text.

nonpenetrant heterozygotes. Converting published formulae to symbols used elsewhere in this book yields

Recurrence risk $= P(1 - P)/2(2 - P - f)$ (Friedman 1985)
Recurrence risk $= P(1 - P)/2(1 - Pf^a)$ (Young 1991)

In Friedman's formula, f is the fitness of all heterozygotes, regardless of their phenotype; in Young's formula, f^a is the fitness of affected (penetrant) heterozygotes, the fitness of unaffected (nonpenetrant) heterozygotes being assumed to be 1.0. When $P = 0.8$ and fitness (either f or f^a) $= 0.7$, these formulae give recurrence risks of

$0.8 * 0.2/2(2 - 0.8 - 0.7) = 0.16/2(0.5) = 0.16 = 16\%$ (Friedman)
$0.8 * 0.2/2(1 - 0.8 * 0.7) = 0.16/2(0.44) = 0.182 = 18.2\%$ (Young)

Why do we have to consider reproductive fitness at all? Because if $P < 1.0$, it is possible to have nonpenetrant heterozygous ancestors, in which case one of the unaffected parents is an obligate heterozygote.

If there are several normal offspring in addition to an affected one born to healthy parents, a Bayesian table can be constructed using the conditional probability of $0.5 + 0.5(1 - P)$ that each child will be normal if one parent is a heterozygote ($4pq$) and 1.0 if both parents are homozygous normal. The probability for the affected child is $0.5P$ when one parent is a heterozygote and $2\mu P$ when both are homozygous normal (or $[\mu + \nu]P$ if the mutation rates are different between the sexes). The recurrence risk will be the posterior risk that one parent is a heterozygote $* 0.5 * P$. Young (1991) derived the following formula using the above procedure

Recurrence risk $= 0.5 * P * [(1 - P)(1 - P/2)^N]/[(1 - P)(1 - P/2)^N + P(1 - f^a)]$

For a family with normal parents and one affected and three healthy children, if $P = 0.8$ and $f^a = 0.7$, the recurrence risk in the next pregnancy would be

Risk $= 0.5 * 0.8 * [0.2(0.6)^3]/[0.2(0.6)^3 + 0.8(0.3)]$
  $= 0.4 * [0.2 * 0.216]/[0.2 * 0.216 + 0.24]$
  $= 0.01728/0.2832 = 0.06102 = 6.1\%$

In Figure 4.5, the presence of a second affected child effectively eliminates new (meiotic) mutation as an explanation. If $P = 1.0$, nonpaternity or germline mosaicism in one parent is a probable explanation. (In both cases, it is assumed that the clinical diagnosis is correct and that we are not dealing with an autosomal recessive form of a disease that exhibits genetic heterogeneity.) If $P < 1.0$, nonpenetrance in a parent can be added to the list of possibilities.

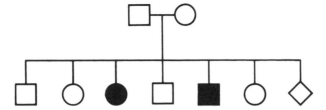

Figure 4.5   A family with an autosomal dominant disease. Several healthy and two affected children have been born to healthy parents, effectively ruling out new meiotic mutations in the affected children. Various explanations are discussed in the text along with the risk of recurrence in the fetus.

The recurrence risk would be 0.5 * P if nonpenetrance is the mechanism, because then one parent would almost certainly be a heterozygote. The recurrence risk would be empirical if germline mosaicism is the explanation (e.g., $P - 1.0$ and parentage established); the actual risk falling somewhere from negligible if the parents were already very unlucky to fertilize two rare mutant gametes up to 0.5 if the parents were lucky to fertilize mostly normal gametes when half were mutant (germline fully heterozygous). In the present case, the only pedigree evidence available suggests that since they already have ²⁄₆ affected children, the recurrence risk will be relatively high. The recurrence risk would be difficult to predict if non-Mendelian mechanisms are operating. If nonpaternity was the explanation for the previous affected children, the recurrence risk is 0.5 * P * #, where # is either 0 or 1 and can be supplied by the mother.

Relevant to all of the preceding discussions is the recently established phenomenon of genomic instability and premutations. In humans, the mechanism was first clearly established for fragile X syndrome and has already been extended to Kennedy disease (X-linked spinal and bulbar muscular atrophy) and myotonic muscular dystrophy. Since myotonic dystrophy is an autosomal dominant disease, this association provides a potential explanation of the phenomenon of anticipation (diseases that get steadily worse over generations). Since the early stages of anticipation might mimic nonpenetrance, then families such as the one shown in Figure 4.5 could be explained as follows: one of the parents has a premutation that although not sufficient to cause symptoms in that parent, predisposes the region to undergo further mutation with a sufficiently high frequency so that some but not all children inheriting that chromosomal region will be affected. The remainder of the children who inherit the at-risk region will have inherited the premutation form of the disease unmodified or modified to a lesser extent than happens during degeneration to the full mutation.

These children, of course, will run the risk of having affected children of their own.

4.2   Autosomal Recessive Inheritance

A recurring question on introductory examinations in human/medical genetics is "If I have a sibling with an autosomal recessive disease, what is my risk of being a carrier?" A Punnett square approach to a carrier versus carrier (Dd versus Dd) cross tells us that the distribution of possible genotypes is DD $\frac{1}{4}$, Dd $\frac{1}{2}$, dd $\frac{1}{4}$, predicting that carrier offspring occur with the probability of $\frac{1}{2}$. We all know, of course, that the answer to the question about my risk is $\frac{2}{3}$, not $\frac{1}{2}$, since the dd genotype can be ignored if I am not clinically affected. This is actually a very simple Bayesian calculation applied to an autosomal condition instead of an X-linked one.

Autosomal recessive inheritance differs fundamentally from X-linked inheritance in that we have to pay much more attention to the males marrying into the pedigree. Figure 4.6 shows the main difference in how the risks are modified by inclusion of the father. In the X-linked case, as we established in chapter 2, the risk is halved each time we move from one female to the next, whether we are going up or down the pedigree. If II-1 is the mother of one healthy son and one son with Duchenne muscular dystrophy and has no prior family history, her risk of being a carrier would be $\frac{1}{2}$ (see Figure 2.5); her mother's risk would be $\frac{1}{4}$, and her sister's risk $\frac{1}{8}$. For comparison, if II-1 in the autosomal recessive case is the grandmother of an affected child, her carrier risk would be $\frac{1}{2}$. Her mother's risk would be $\frac{1}{4}$, as in the X-linked pedigree, but her father's carrier risk also has to be considered and is also $\frac{1}{4}$. Her sister's risk is half of their mother's risk ($\frac{1}{8}$) plus half of their father's risk ($\frac{1}{8}$). The combined risk of $\frac{1}{4}$ is therefore twice as high as in an X-linked condition, where mothers and fathers have to be treated very differently.

All of the foregoing arguments assume that autosomal recessive mutations are ancient and that new mutations occur extremely rarely. This assumption was based mostly in ignorance, and I think that it will come under increasing scrutiny as direct mutation testing becomes available for progressively more diseases (see, for example, White et al. 1991). Recent revelations pertaining to non-Mendelian inheritance (uniparental disomy, in particular) will also probably force a reevaluation of the wisdom of assuming that both parents of a child with an autosomal recessive condition are obligate carriers of the disease.

In Figure 4.7, the two affected children have metachromatic leuko-

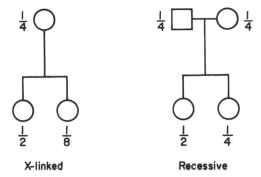

X-linked   **Recessive**

Figure 4.6   Pedigrees that illustrate the difference in risk between siblings in families with isolated cases of X-linked recessive and autosomal recessive diseases. In both families, assume that the daughter II-1 has a carrier risk of 1/2 because of an affected descendant. The risk that her sister is a carrier differs significantly depending upon the mode of inheritance.

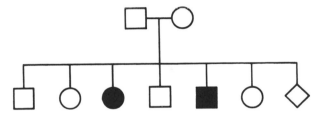

Figure 4.7   A family with autosomal recessive metachromatic leukodystrophy (MLD). Although the Mendelian risk for the fetus is straightforward (1/4), biochemical testing results are complicated because many different mechanisms can reduce enzyme levels. As discussed in the text not all of these mechanisms cause disease, so caution and a thorough understanding of the pathogenesis of the disease are very important.

dystrophy (MLD), an autosomal recessive inborn error of metabolism resulting in deficiency of the enzyme arylsulfatase A. The parents are expecting their seventh child and, facing a ¼ recurrence risk, opt for prenatal diagnosis for MLD. The biochemical genetics laboratory studies the prenatal sample and finds negligible enzyme activity. Fortunately, they also had obtained samples from the rest of the family and tested them before issuing a report stating that the fetus will be affected.

They found that I-1, II-2, II-3, II-5, and II-6 had negligible activity, apparently meaning that they should all be affected, and that I-2, II-1, and II-4 had approximately 50% activity, consistent with being carriers of the disease. Nobody had normal (100%) levels of the enzyme. This family has two types of mutation in the arylsulfatase A gene: one causing true deficiency of arylsulfatase A and another causing "pseudodeficiency" of arylsulfatase A. We now know that "true" mutations result in a defective or absent enzyme, whereas "pseudo"-mutations result in instability of the mRNA (poly(A) site mutation), which nevertheless encodes a perfectly normal polypeptide. The "pseudo" allele allows the synthesis of very low levels of normal polypeptide, which on a simple enzyme assay mimics "true" mutations, which allow the synthesis of larger quantities of inactive polypeptide. The difference clinically is that when stressed in vivo by high levels of substrate, enough enzyme is produced from the "pseudo" allele to permit good health even when it is present in homozygous form or (worse still) in compound heterozygosity with a "true" MLD mutation. "True" mutations yield nonfunctional (or no) enzymes under any circumstance. The healthy father, I-1, in this family was a compound heterozygote for a true mutation and the pseudodeficiency mutation; his wife was a heterozygous carrier of a true mutation only. II-2 and II-6 are compound heterozygotes who inherited the pseudodeficiency allele from their father (which ensures their good health) and the true mutation from their mother. II-3 and II-5 inherited true mutations from both parents and are therefore affected by MLD. II-1 and II-4, with approximately enzyme 50% activity, inherited the pseudodeficiency allele from their father and a normal allele from their mother. The fetus, III-7, therefore, requires urgent clarification of whether its negligible enzyme activity is due to homozygosity for true mutations or to compound heterozygosity: in the former case, it will be affected; in the latter, healthy. Fortunately, additional biochemical (sulfatide-loading assay) and molecular tests discriminate between these two possibilities.

This example was included because, although pseudodeficiency of arylsulfatase A is now well characterized for MLD, poly(A) mutations could theoretically cause similar difficulties in the analysis of any diseases due to enzyme deficiencies. The frequency of heterozygous carriers of the arylsulfatase A pseudodeficiency allele is approximately 1 in 7 people, so it is inevitable that a proportion of MLD families where both parents are carriers of true mutations will also have at least one pseudodeficiency allele as well. Since arylsulfatase A activity can also be reduced or absent due to deficiency of activator proteins or due to multiple sulfatase deficiency, the importance of a good theoretical knowledge of the system being studied cannot be overemphasized.

In Figure 4.8, the consultants are E and F, who are first cousins. Consanguinity is an important issue in autosomal recessive conditions, because it provides a mechanism to generate homozygotes for a rare allele. If a common ancestor was a carrier of an autosomal recessive

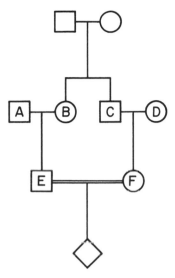

Figure 4.8 A consanguineous marriage between first cousins. Their unborn child has a higher risk of an autosomal recessive disease than the general population if either or both great-grandparents are carriers, but a lower risk if neither great-grandparent is a carrier (requiring both of the individuals marrying into the pedigree, A and D, to be carriers).

disease and both members of the consanguineous couple inherited the same allele from that ancestor (probability $\frac{1}{8}$), their risk of having an affected child is much higher than the risk for two unrelated people from a randomly mating population (risk $= q^2$ where $q =$ frequency of the deleterious recessive allele). What is the exact risk for first cousins? This is a complex series of different scenarios. First, the cousins, E and F, could have 0, 1, or 2 carrier grandparents. If one or both grandparents are carriers, multiple permutations allow us to end with two recessive alleles in the fetus; if neither grandparent is a carrier, it is still possible to have an affected child if both A and D are carriers (in which case there is technically a decreased risk through being first cousins). Fortunately, there is a formula that, for first cousins, gives the risk of having a child affected with a recessive disease as

$$q(1 + 15q)/16 \qquad \text{(Maynard-Smith et al. 1961)}$$

If the cousins are concerned about cystic fibrosis and we assume an allele frequency of either 0.025 or 0.020 ($\frac{1}{40}$ or $\frac{1}{50}$), this formula would give risks of 0.002148 ($\frac{1}{465}$) and 0.001625 ($\frac{1}{615}$), which are approximately 3.4 and 4.0 times greater than if they were unrelated, 0.000625 and 0.000400 ($\frac{1}{1,600}$ and $\frac{1}{2,500}$).

5

Introduction to
DNA Polymorphisms

Polymorphism means occurring in different forms. The hereditary nature of genetic polymorphisms has been at least partially understood for thousands of years. As one example, there are pedigrees and breeding records of horses recorded in ancient Egyptian hieroglyphics. Similarly, the hereditary nature and even the exact mode of transmission of some human diseases have been recognized for thousands of years. Ancient Jewish law permitted the exemption for circumcision of further sons if one had bled severely following the procedure, thereby recognizing the familial nature of hemophilia. Furthermore, sons of the mother's sisters were exempted, but if the father remarried, any sons from the second marriage did not have this exemption (Milunsky 1992, p. 90), which surely demonstrates an understanding of the existence of carrier females but the lack of male-to-male transmission of an X-linked disorder. Similar ancient religious proscriptions against incest or the marriage of close relatives also could be taken to imply at least some degree of understanding of the genetic significance and potential consequences of inbreeding.

Ancient observations, however, were limited to phenotypically obvious characteristics. It was not until laboratory science permitted the differentiation between isoforms of proteins, blood groups, etc., that the number of polymorphisms available (Roychoudhury and Nei 1988) for the study of human linkage groups became sufficient to make this anything other than searching for a needle in a haystack. The several discoveries leading to the realization that variations in DNA sequence might lead to alterations in restriction endonuclease recognition sequences that were (*a*) codominantly inherited, (*b*) easily detected, and (*c*) very frequent offered previously unimaginable possibilities for the study of human linkage groups.

Consider two sets of DNA sequences:

ACGGAATAGGCCC<u>C</u>CAATCTAAAGCCCGTGAAGGTAAACC
ACGGAATAGGCCC<u>T</u>CAATCTAAAGCCCGTGAAGGTAAACC

and

ACGGAATAGGCCCCCAA<u>TCTA</u>AAGCCCGTGAAGGTAAACC
ACGGAATAGGCCCCCAA<u>TCGA</u>AAGCCCGTGAAGGTAAACC

In both cases, the underlined region contains a point mutation. In the latter case, the mutation of the underlined TCTA sequence to TCGA generates a recognition sequence for the restriction site recognized by the enzyme Taq I; in the former case, the point mutation neither creates nor destroys a restriction site. (Most restriction endonucleases used in diagnostic laboratories recognize palindromic 4, 5, or 6 base-pair sequences and cleave the DNA within that sequence.) The difference between the two in effect on health may or may not be important, but from a laboratory point of view, the latter change, which creates a new restriction site, is very much easier to discover than the former change, which would be found only by DNA sequence analysis. If the mutation in the restriction site is also the cause of the disease, we have a direct and relatively simple test to detect the presence or absence of the disease-causing allele. If the restriction site mutation is not the cause of the disease, it is called a *polymorphism* (this term is usually taken to imply that it is a harmless variant). The utility of the polymorphism in gene mapping or in the study of genetic risks depends upon how frequently the two (or more) different alleles occur in the population. If it is very rare, sometimes called a *private variant,* it will generally be of use only in the study of members of a single family. If it is found fairly frequently in the general population, it is a useful *restriction fragment length polymorphism* (RFLP). Two numbers can be calculated to give a general guide to how useful an RFLP is likely to be in linkage studies. The heterozygosity (het) is the frequency of heterozygotes expected in the general population under Hardy-Weinberg equilibrium (which is an indication of, but not necessarily the same as, the frequency of heterozygotes in the specific family that you are about to study). The polymorphism information content (PIC) is similar but subtracts the probability of uninformative matings (such as child and parents all heterozygous for the same alleles where the contribution of each parent to the child cannot be resolved) from the overall heterozygosity. Het and PIC are equal for X-linked loci where the maternal contribution can always be resolved.

RFLPs are a convenient way of detecting variations in DNA sequence; however, the variation does not actually need to coincide with a restriction site. There are many cases of structural modification (insertion/deletion) polymorphisms that affect the distance between restriction sites and thus create an RFLP. The first extremely useful class to be described in detail was the *variable number of tandem repeat* (VNTR) polymorphisms, where a repetitive region of DNA was repeated a variable number of times. The more times the unit was repeated, the further apart any restriction sites spanning this region would be pushed. The great advantage of this type of polymorphism over the earlier described biallelic RFLPs was that there were a large number of potential alleles. For a biallelic system, with alleles A and B, there are only three potential genotypes, AA, AB, and BB. For a VNTR-type polymorphism with, for example, ten possible alleles, A–J, there are 55 potential genotypes (AA, AB, AC, AD, . . . , JH, JI, JJ). For N different alleles, the number of different genotypes is the sum of the series $N + (N - 1) + (N - 2) + (N - 3)$, etc., decreasing until we reach a value of 1. The formula that gives the number of different genotypes from N different alleles is $N(N + 1)/2$. If there are a large number of different potential genotypes, the chances of being homozygous obviously diminish, which means that the chances of being uninformative for linkage studies also diminishes. The other advantage of VNTRs is that the same variation can be detected as an RFLP by several different restriction enzymes (any that has sites a suitable distance away from each end of the repetitive region), whereas biallelic enzyme site polymorphisms are detected by only that specific enzyme or its isoschizomers (enzymes from a different bacterium that recognize the same sequence). This last point makes biallelic enzyme site polymorphisms harder to detect originally because they will be missed unless a "screening blot" prepared with DNA cut with the correct enzyme is used. Also the enzyme may be very expensive, and for VNTRs it may be possible to substitute a cheaper enzyme.

Another class of polymorphism, which is really the equivalent of miniature VNTR polymorphisms, is the microsatellite polymorphisms. These contain repetitive units of a short, simple sequence such as CA (called CA repeats, or TG repeats by those who refer to the complementary strand). Other examples of short repeat motifs are $(AAT)_n$, $(AGC)_n$, $(AATG)_n$, $(ACAG)_n$, and $(AGAT)_n$ or $(TCTA)_n$ (the last has been known for more than ten years in snakes as a BK_m repeat and represents an example of something well known in other species being applied to humans only after a substantial lag). The locus involved in fragile X syndrome is highly polymorphic in the normal population, with a repeat motif of $(CGG)_n$ occasionally interspersed with AGG. In the disease state, this CGG motif undergoes amplification and is present in hundreds of copies.

These and similar repetitive polymorphisms have been found very widely dispersed throughout the human genome, almost all are easily detected by PCR-based methods, and their discovery marked a major step forward in the project to develop a finely detailed linkage map of the human genome.

To return to the original examples of DNA sequence given above, the first point mutation did not modify a restriction site nor did it modify the overall length of the DNA molecule by insertion or deletion. This change needs to be identified as a sequence variant. This can, of course, be done by sequencing that region of DNA, but that is expensive. If the variant is fairly frequent in the population, it may be worth constructing *allele-specific oligonucleotides* (ASOs) to act as probes for the one of the two potential sequences at that point (one will form a perfect double helix, and the other will have a mismatch; the inverse will apply when the second ASO is used). Many other methods are currently being developed to allow the rapid and cost-effective identification of point mutations that do not modify restriction enzyme sites. A partial list of some of the methods and acronyms given to these procedures is given here, along with whether they can normally identify previously unknown mutations (screen) or only previously characterized mutations for which the surrounding DNA sequence is known (known). Any procedure that can identify unknown mutations can obviously also be used to identify known ones (but it may not be the most efficient or cost-effective).

ASO	allele-specific oligonucleotides	(known)
CC	chemical cleavage	(screen)
DGGE	denaturing gradient gel electrophoresis	(screen)
	allele-specific ligation	(known)
PASA	PCR amplification of specific alleles	(known)
	sequence analysis	(screen)
SSCP	single-strand conformational polymorphisms	(screen)

In the sections on Bayesian calculations, the objective was to calculate the probability that someone was a carrier of a genetic disease, using the reproductive history of his or her family. The conditional probabilities were limited to the ratio between the probability of having a normal son if you are a carrier of the disease and the probability of having a normal son if you are not a carrier of the disease. The ratio between these two hypotheses was never very high (in fact, could not exceed 2:1) because it represents a random pick between two possibilities.

When DNA markers are used in studies of genetic linkage, it becomes possible to know or infer that a specific chromosome or chromosomal locus was inherited, that is, the selection is no longer random. Under these circumstances, it is possible to generate much higher ratios between carrier and noncarrier columns. If recombination is known to occur between two adjacent loci with a frequency of 1% (that is an average of one per 100 meioses), then the knowledge of what was inherited at one locus will have very strong predictive value regarding what was inherited at the second, linked locus. The Greek letter θ (theta) is used in genetics to denote recombination fraction and is expressed as a number between 0.00 and 0.50, indicative of 0 to 50% recombination. 50% recombination ($\theta = 0.50$) is the theoretical maximum because even if two loci are on different chromosomes, they will be inherited together half of the time (50%) by chance.

The terms *phase-known* and *phase-unknown* are used to refer to whether or not we are certain of the arrangement of the various alleles at both loci in a person. Let us assume that there are two linked loci, A and B, and that locus A has two alleles, termed A1 and A2, and locus B has two alleles, termed B1 and B2. If a man is a double heterozygote (A1,A2;B1,B2) and we have studied both of his parents, we may be able to establish unequivocally that A1 and B1 were inherited together from his father and A2 and B2 were inherited together from his mother. If this is so, then we know that the A1 and B1 alleles are on the same chromosome in him and are said to be in coupling. A1 and B2 are on opposite chromosomes and are said to be in repulsion. We can write this as A1-B1/A2-B2 to indicate that he is phase-known and that A1 and B1 are in coupling (as are A2 and B2 on the other chromosome). Without studying his parents, we would have no evidence to prove that the phase of the alleles at these loci is not A1-B2/A2-B1.

Once we have established the correct phase in a person, the only way that alleles that were in coupling can become in repulsion is through the process of recombination. Nonrecombinant offspring will have a frequency of $1 - \theta$ and recombinant offspring will have a frequency of θ. When one of the loci involved is a disease locus, the knowledge of what allele at the test locus was inherited through a phase-known meiosis is very useful in predictive calculations.

In Figure 5.1, the grandfather, I-1, has an X-linked recessive disease, so his daughter, II-1, is an obligate carrier of this disease. His granddaughter, III-1, has a 50% prior risk of being a carrier. To try to resolve her status, an analysis has been performed on the family group, using

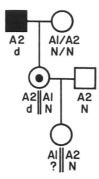

Figure 5.1   A phase-known pedigree in which the grandfather has an X-linked recessive disease. The marker locus A has alleles A1 and A2 and recombines with
the disease locus in 5% of meioses (θ = 0.05). The disease locus has a recessive
allele d (disease) and a dominant allele N (normal). The *sloping lines* separating
the alleles at each locus in I-2 indicate that she is phase-unknown; the *continuous vertical lines* drawn between the alleles at both loci in II-1 indicate that she
is phase-known with the A2-d haplotype on one X chromosome (the paternal
one) and the A1-N haplotype on her maternal X chromosome.

a DNA marker that recombines with the disease 5% of the time (θ =
0.05). Since the disease-causing mutation and allele A2 at the marker
locus are both known to be on the grandfather's single X chromosome,
the phase in II-1 is known to be A2-d/A1-N because we know that I-1
has to pass on the A2-d combination intact (there is no possibility of
recombination for true X-linked loci in 46,XY males). III-1 has inherited A2-N from her father, and, by subtraction of his contribution,
A1-? from her mother. She will be a carrier if ? = d and a noncarrier
if ? = N. Since A1 was coupled to N in her mother, III-1 will be a
carrier only if recombination occurred during meiosis in her mother.
The probability that recombination occurred is θ, which in this example is 0.05 (5%), which is therefore her risk of being a carrier.

One further point is *absolutely essential* to the interpretation of DNA
tests using linked markers. The result of the DNA test (maternal A1)
would be exactly the same if III-1 is a carrier or if she is a noncarrier.
The recombination fraction of θ = 0.05 is an empirical number derived
from population studies. It is absolutely impossible to tell from the
marker result whether or not recombination occurred *this time*. If such
a determination were possible, directors of DNA laboratories would
be in the happy position of always reporting 0% or 100% risk. This is
not the case, and the quoted risk of 5% indicates that although probability is on her side, noncarrier status cannot be guaranteed.

Having taken care to stress the cautionary side of these probabilities,
let us look instead at what has happened to the noncarrier:carrier

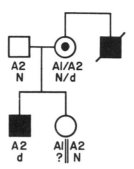

Figure 5.2   A family with an X-linked recessive disease that has been studied with a DNA marker (locus A) that recombines with the disease in 5% of meioses (θ = 0.05). The mother, I-2, is phase-unknown because we have not studied her parents. We can calculate the probability of each of the two possible phases in her (A1-d/A2-N or A1-N/A2-d), using the premise that her affected son is much more likely to be nonrecombinant than recombinant between the disease and marker loci when θ = 0.05. The probability that her daughter is a carrier can then be calculated for each potential maternal phase as shown in Table 5.1.

ratios in this case. Without the DNA test, III-1 had a 50% risk of being a carrier. Based upon her genotype at the marker locus, we now predict that she has a 5% risk of being a carrier (carrier = 0.05, noncarrier = 0.95). This is a nineteenfold improvement (0.5/0.5 = 1.00, 0.95/0.05 = 19.00). If we compare this with the Bayesian risks in chapter 2, this single DNA test has a stronger influence on her carrier risk than if she had four normal sons (0.5 noncarrier/0.03125 carrier = 16.00). The column ratios resulting from DNA tests tend to be much greater than those from other types of test.

Under circumstances where it has not been possible to determine phase with certainty because we have been unable to study the person's parents, it is frequently possible to infer the phase from the study of offspring, on the assumption that arrangements noted in offspring reflect the arrangement in the parent unless recombination occurred. In such instances, all potential phases must be considered, and the probability of each being the correct one is calculated by what is essentially a Bayesian calculation performed in reverse. Given that a heterozygous female who is a carrier of hemophilia A has an affected son with the genotype A2-dis, what is the probability that her genotype is A2-dis/A1-NOR (1 − θ, because the son would be nonrecombinant), or what is the probability that her genotype is A2-NOR/A1-dis (θ, because he would be recombinant). If she had other sons, it would be possible to obtain even stronger evidence in support of one particular phase being the correct one in her, since the ratio would become (1

Table 5.1 Calculation of the risk that II-2 in Figure 5.2 is a carrier of the X-linked recessive disorder using an RFLP linked at $\theta = 0.05$

	Phase in I-2			
	A1-N/A2-d		A1-d/A2-N	
Prior probability	0.5		0.5	
II-1 = A2-d	0.95		0.05	
Posterior probability	0.95		0.05	
II-2 =	Carrier	Noncarrier	Carrier	Noncarrier
Maternal A1	0.05	0.95	0.95	0.05
Joint probability	0.0475	0.9025	0.0475	0.0025

Total carrier = 0.0475 + 0.0475 = 0.095
Total noncarrier = 0.9025 + 0.0025 = 0.905

Notes: A1 and A2 are alternative alleles of the RFLP; d = recessive disease-causing allele, N = dominant normal allele.

$- \theta)^2$ to θ^2 for two sons, $(1 - \theta)^3$ to θ^3 for three sons, and so forth. When considering the risk to her next child, it is necessary to calculate the risk to the child from each potential maternal phase and then to determine the cumulative risk by adding the individual risks obtained for each phase.

In Figure 5.2, the carrier mother, I-2, is phase-unknown because we have not been able to study her parents to determine the origin of each allele. We can nevertheless conclude that it is much more likely that her affected son is nonrecombinant $(1 - \theta)$ than recombinant (θ), in which case, we can assume that the phase in her that would permit the generation of his genotype without recombination is the more likely. In Figure 5.1, we knew the mother's phase and used that information to determine the relative probabilities of her daughter's two possible genotypes. In Figure 5.2, we can do the exact reverse: use the son's known genotype to determine the relative probabilities of his mother's two possible phases. We can then calculate the probability that the daughter, II-2, is a carrier for each maternal phase (Table 5.1).

Figure 5.3 shows diagrammatically the difference between a phase-known meiosis and a phase-inferred meiosis with respect to the risk that the next child will have the same X-linked disease. Assume that the mother is an obligate carrier and that θ is known to be 0.05. In the phase-known portion of the diagram, the phase in the mother is known

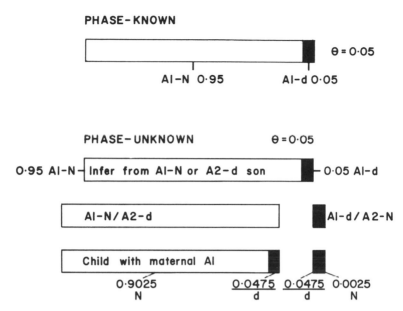

Figure 5.3   A diagram to illustrate the difference between phase-known and phase-unknown meioses. Marker locus A (alleles A1 and A2) recombines with the disease locus (alleles d and N) in 5% of meioses ($\theta = 0.05$). In the *upper part* of the diagram assume that a phase-known A1-N/A2-d mother has passed the A1 allele to a male fetus. Since $\theta = 0.05$, it is much more likely that recombination did not occur between the marker and disease loci (leaving the A1-N haplotype intact) and that the fetus will be normal (probability $= 1 - \theta = 0.95$ represented by the *white part of the bar*). For the A1 allele to be associated with the disease allele in an A1-d haplotype requires recombination (probability $= \theta = 0.05$ represented by the *black part of the bar*). The *lower part* of the diagram is split into three lines. The carrier mother is phase-unknown A1/A2, d/N. If she has either a normal son with genotype A1-N or an affected son with genotype A2-d, we can infer that the phase in her is more likely to be A1-N/A2-d (shown by the *long white bar on the second line*) than A1-d/A2-N (shown by the *shorter black bar*). If she has a second child who inherits allele A1 from her, the probability that it will be A1-N is shown by the *white bars on the third line* under each of the potential maternal phases shown on the *second line*, and the probability that it will be A1-d is shown by the *black bar* under each potential maternal phase. The total risk would be 0.0475 + 0.0475 or 0.0905 (9.5%) by a calculation very similar to the one shown in Table 5.1.

to be A1-NOR/A2-dis. The risk that the next child will inherit the disease allele will be 0.05 (θ) if allele A1 was inherited (represented by the shaded area) and the chance that it will be normal will be 0.95 ($1 - \theta$, represented by the unshaded area). Since the mother is phase-known, there is no chance of our being misled even if her first son has the genotype A1-dis, since we would know that he was a recombinant.

In the second case, however, we are using the premise that the earlier child is nonrecombinant to determine the most probable phase in the mother, and then we apply that assumption to the calculation of risk for the next child. Since an assumption has to be made, the potential for error is obviously greater, and this is reflected in the final risk. If her first son has the genotype A2-dis, we can infer that her phase is either A1-NOR/A2-dis (probability of 0.95, represented by the unshaded area) or A1-dis/A2-NOR (probability of 0.05, represented by the shaded area). For each of these two potential maternal phases, the probability that the next child who inherited a maternal A1 allele also inherited the disease can be calculated to be $0.95 * 0.05 + 0.05 * 0.95$, which represents the probability that A1 is coupled to the normal allele in the mother (first child nonrecombinant), multiplied by the probability that through recombination it becomes coupled to the mutant allele in the next child, plus the probability that A1 is coupled to the disease in the mother (first child recombinant), multiplied by the probability that it remains coupled to the disease allele in the next child (no recombination). Alternatively, if the second child inherits the other marker allele (relative to the first affected child), the second child will be affected if either is recombinant ($2 * \theta[1 - \theta] = 2 * 0.05 * 0.95$, total $= 0.095$), but unaffected if neither is recombinant ($[1 - \theta]^2 = 0.95 * 0.95$) or both are recombinant ($\theta^2 = 0.05 * 0.05$, total 0.905).

Figure 5.4 shows the same principles as a funnel diagram. The large funnel represents the more probable phase and its significant constriction the fact that a recombination event would be required to generate an affected child (4.75% total risk). The small funnel represents the less probable phase, and the minor constriction the fact that no recombination is required to generate an affected child (also a 4.75% risk).

When two DNA markers are available that are known to be located on opposite sides of the disease-causing locus, we have what are known as flanking markers. The identification of flanking markers is always a very important step in the development of molecular tests for a genetic disease for the following reason. If $\theta = 0.10$, a single marker locus will recombine with the disease locus 10% of the time, which is not very satisfactory; however, if there is a second marker locus on the other side of the disease locus, let us say also at $\theta = 0.10$, the second marker will tell us that a recombination event took place except in the rare case of a second recombination event taking place in the same meiosis between the disease locus and the second marker locus. Since the meiotic crossovers would represent independent events, the probability of both occurring simultaneously (a double crossover) is the product of their individual probabilities (in this case, $0.1 * 0.1 = 0.01$). This principle is illustrated in Figure 5.5.

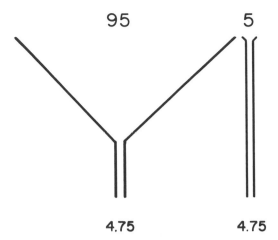

Figure 5.4   The same principle as in the lower part of Fig. 5.3 shown as a funnel diagram (θ = 0.05). The *tops* of the funnels represent the probabilities of the two maternal phases (0.95 or 95% and 0.05 or 5%); the *bottoms* of the funnels represent the probability that the next child will be affected (0.0475 or 4.75% for each phase). The *major constriction* of the funnel on the *left* indicates that, although this is the more likely phase in the mother, a recombination event would be necessary to generate an affected child. The *minor constriction* of the funnel on the *right* indicates that, although this is the less likely phase in the mother, no recombination is required to generate an affected child.

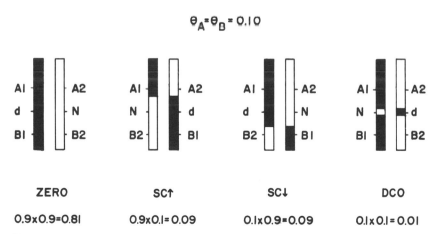

Figure 5.5   The probabilities of no crossovers, single crossovers above or below the disease locus (*SC* ↑ and *SC* ↓), and double crossovers (*DCO*) within an region defined by locus A—(θ_A = 0.10)—disease locus—(θ_B = 0.10)—locus B.

PARENT PHASE-KNOWN AI-N-BI/A2-d-B2

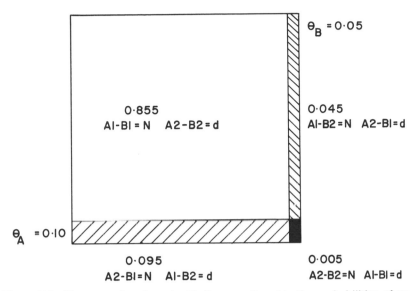

Figure 5.6 The *area of each rectangle* is proportional to the probabilities of no crossovers (*white*), single crossovers (*hatched*), or double crossovers (*black*) among the offspring of a phase-known A1-N-B1/A2-d-B2 parent. An A2-?-B2 haplotype found in the offspring has the following probabilities: the ratio of d:N = 0.855:0.005. An A2-?-B1 haplotype would have the ratio d:N = 0.045:0.095.

The mathematics of the same principle are shown graphically in Figure 5.6. In this example, marker locus A is assumed to recombine with the disease locus 10% of the time (represented by the hatched strip across the bottom of the square) and flanking marker locus B, 5% of the time (represented by the hatched strip along the right edge). The unshaded area represents the probability that neither will recombine, and the black area at the lower right corner the probability that both will recombine in the same meiosis (a double crossover event). Single crossover events will be identified by the fact that they yield a different genotype in the offspring from that present in the phase-known parent. If a single crossover can be eliminated as a possibility by inspection of the genotype (e.g., finding an A1-B1 genotype), the risk of being affected can be determined by comparing the area of the two remaining rectangles. In this case there is a 0.855/0.86 = 99.4% probability that N is sandwiched between the A1 and B1 markers (no crossover) and a 0.005/0.86 = 0.6% probability that d is sandwiched between these markers (a double crossover). The risk is much less satisfactory if a single crossover is known to have occurred by virtue of finding an A1-B2 or A2-B1 genotype in the offspring, but this is still very much better than the situation without the flanking marker, because without it you would not know that the crossover event had occurred. An A1-B2 genotype would have the following risks: $0.045/0.14 = 32.1\%$ normal (A nonrecombinant, B recombinant) or $0.095/0.14 = 67.9\%$ affected (A recombinant, B nonrecombinant). (Logical check: B2 was associated with the disease in the phase-known parent, and the B locus recombines less frequently than the A locus; therefore, a genotype containing B2 should have a greater than 50% risk of being affected.) This is not much better than the 50% risk without DNA testing, but it is safer than the 5% or 10% that would have been quoted using only one marker and relying on the probability that a crossover did not occur.

In all of the preceding discussion, even though the phase is not necessarily known, we have assumed that the recombination fraction, θ, is known accurately. To keep the horse before the cart, however, before we can proceed to the main examples of how known recombination fractions between DNA markers and disease loci can be used to predict genotype at the disease locus, we need to see how the recombination fractions are determined.

In an experimental organism, the determination of recombination fractions is easy; phase-known crosses are "arranged" and thousands of offspring are typed, so an accurate count of, say, 50 recombinant and 4,950 nonrecombinant offspring are discovered among a total of 5,000. In this case, the recombination fraction is 50/5,000, or 1%. This approach has several ethical and technical problems in human genetics.

Human recombination fractions are estimated by linkage analysis, which is a type of gene mapping. In linkage analysis, θ is the unknown variable to be computed from the consideration of the likelihood of finding all the particular (known) genotypes distributed among the various members of a family. Risk calculation is a related process for which θ must be known with a fair degree of accuracy so that the unknown variable can be set as the genotype of a selected member of the family.

6

Statistical Approaches to
Gene Mapping

6.1 Lod Scores

The relative positions of loci on the same chromosome (syntenic = same thread) are estimated by calculating the frequency with which recombination occurs between them. If recombination occurs in less than 50% of a statistically large number of meioses, the loci are not segregating independently (as expected by Mendel's second law) and are said to be linked. The degree of linkage may be expressed in several ways: (a) percentage recombination (%); (b) map distances (in centi-Morgans, or cM) where 1 cM ≈ 1% recombination (although this relationship becomes nonlinear with increasing distance; see the discussion of mapping functions at the end of this section; or (c) recombination fractions (Greek letter theta), where $\theta = 0.5$ for 50% recombination or $\theta = 0.15$ for 15% recombination. Linked loci are always syntenic, but the converse is not necessarily true: loci on the same chromosome will segregate independently when $\theta = 0.5$.

Since large numbers of offspring cannot be studied in single human families, mathematical methods have been devised for estimating both the degree of linkage (θ) and the likelihood (odds), for any potential value of θ, that the loci are linked rather than unlinked (lod score = *logarithm* of the *odds*: symbol = Z). A negative lod score for that value of θ is evidence that the hypothesis is incorrect and that the spatial arrangement of the loci is not such that that value for θ is true; a positive lod score (in particular, a large positive lod score) supports the hypothesis that the loci are linked. The most probable genetic distance between the two loci is determined by plotting the recombination fraction θ versus the lod score calculated for each value of θ: the value of θ at which the highest (peak) lod score is obtained is the most likely value for the recombination fraction between the two loci. This value of θ is designated with a circumflex ^ ($\hat{\theta}$). The peak lod score at that value of θ is designated $Z(\hat{\theta})$ or frequently just $\hat{Z}$. The lod scores can be calculated manually (see below), but they are usually calculated by computer programs. Some programs are written primarily for linkage analysis, such as LIPED (Ott 1974) or LINKAGE (Lathrop and Lalouel 1984); others are written primarily for constructing genetic maps, such as MAPMAKER (Lander et al. 1987), or primarily for risk calculation, such as SCHESIS (Round 1989). To some extent, most of these programs perform some or most of the other functions. I have used the risk-calculating program SCHESIS quite frequently because it is "user friendly" and because it provides an easy means of editing data, so it can be used for "what-if" modeling in complex situations. It also contains a plotting function that draws the pedigree on the computer screen (Round 1992), which is extremely useful for checking the accuracy of the data entered and also provides a printed record of the pedigree to store with the numerical analysis.

To help us understand the theory of lod scores and to see how they are calculated, we will perform some sample calculations, progressing from a family with one child to a family with five children. Although the lod scores in these situations would still be too low to be considered significant, the general principles can be understood. The first example is an autosomal dominant disorder with 100% penetrance at birth (D = affected, d = not affected) and a DNA marker (RFLP type detecting the presence or absence of a restriction site) with two alleles, A1 and A2. For each family, assume that the grandfather was affected (D/d) and had DNA alleles A1/A1 (homozygous), that the unaffected grandmother (d/d) had DNA alleles A2/A2 (homozygous), that the affected mother (D/d) had DNA alleles A1/A2, and that her husband was unaffected (d/d) and had DNA alleles (A1/A1). Since the affected mother inherited the disease from her father, if the disease and the DNA marker are linked, her phase is known to be A1D/A2d, since she inherited allele A1 from her father and allele A2 from her unaffected mother. Any of her children who is affected and who has the A1 marker will be nonrecombinant (NR) and any of her children who is affected and has the A2 marker will be recombinant (R). Since the children must all inherit A1 and d from their unaffected father, the possible genotypes and phases in the offspring are (maternal chromosome shown first)

A1D/A1d	nonrecombinant	(NR)	affected	(AFF)
A2d/A1d	nonrecombinant	(NR)	normal	(NOR)
A1d/A1d	recombinant	(R)	normal	(NOR)
A2D/A1d	recombinant	(R)	affected	(AFF)

If the loci are inseparably linked at $\theta = 0.0$, the probability of having an NR child is 1.000. If the loci are linked at $\theta = 0.1$, the probability of having a NR child is 0.900 and an R child, 0.100. If the loci are not linked ($\theta = 0.5$), the probability of having an NR child is the same as that of having an R child (both 0.500) (Figure 6.1 and Table 6.1). This is the weakest possible evidence of linkage. If the child instead is A1d/A1d NOR R (family B), the calculation would become as shown in Table 6.2. A lod score of $-\infty$ (the log of zero) means that the situation is impossible (for example, recombination between loci linked at a recombination fraction of zero). A negative lod score is evidence that for that particular recombination fraction the loci are unlikely to be linked.

Adding a second NR child (Table 6.3) has increased the lod score by 0.3 when $\theta = 0$, which is the same as saying that the odds in favor of linkage have increased by a factor of 2 (log 2 = 0.301). Every NR child doubles the odds at $\theta = 0$, which makes sense when one considers that there is a twofold difference between an event with a probability of 1.0 (coinheritance when tightly linked) and an event with a probability of 0.5 (coinheritance when unlinked) (Table 6.4). This also tells us that to achieve a lod score of 6 would require 6/0.3 or 20 phase-known meioses when $\theta = 0$ and more than 20 meioses when $\theta > 0$ and the linked:unlinked ratio decreases from 2.0 toward 1.0. Those familiar with the polymerase chain reaction might recognize similar logic applied to a different setting: 20 cycles gives approximately a millionfold amplification, because $2^{20} \approx 10^6$ or 20 log 2 $\approx$ 6.0. If the doubling efficiency is less than 100%, more than 20 cycles will be needed to attain this desired degree of amplification.

The presence of a single recombinant offspring (Table 6.5) rules out the possibility of linkage at a recombination fraction of $\hat{\theta} = 0.0$. The maximum lod score for this family ($\hat{Z} = 0.418$) actually occurs at $\hat{\theta} = 0.2$ (but don't believe it—prove it by calculating values on either side of 0.2, such as 0.19 and 0.21). (This is the expected result, since a simple head count of one recombinant out of a total of five offspring represents 20% recombination.)

One very important advantage of lod scores is that they represent the logarithms of independent probabilities. Since independent probabilities are combined by multiplication, this can be achieved by adding

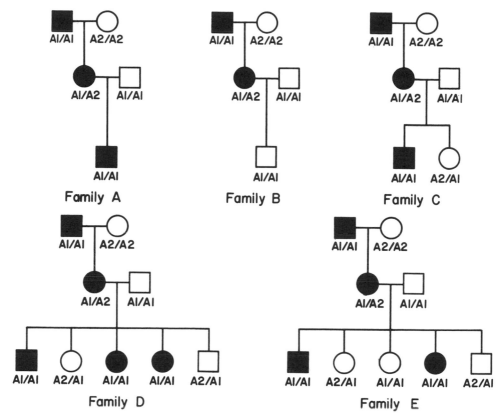

Figure 6.1   Five families that will be used to illustrate the basics of how recombination fractions and lod scores are calculated. Assume that all families have the same fully penetrant autosomal dominant disorder. Marker locus A has two alleles, A1 and A2. We want to determine the recombination fraction between the marker and disease loci. Study of the first generation permits us to determine that if the marker locus is linked to the disease locus, female II-1 in each family is phase-known A1-D/A2-n. The likelihood of linkage between these loci is calculated in Tables 6.1 to 6.6.

lod scores from different families for each value of θ. The total lod score for these five families is obtained in Table 6.6. These values for the total lod score are equal to twice the values for a 6NR:1R family of seven children, since combining two families, each with 6NR:1R, represents the same number of meioses (14) (12NR:2R) as the above families A–E. The results for two families, one with 7NR:0R and the other with 5NR:2R, should also be the same—try it.

Two recombinant children out of a total of fourteen offspring should give a peak lod score at a recombination fraction of $^2/_{14}$ or $\hat{\theta} = 0.14$

Table 6.1   Calculation of lod score for family A in Figure 6.1, given that the child is nonrecombinant

	Linked					Unlinked
$\theta = 0.0$	0.1	0.2	0.3	0.4	0.5
Assuming loci are linked	1.000	0.900	0.800	0.700	0.600	0.500
Assuming loci are unlinked						0.500
Ratio linked : unlinked	2.000	1.800	1.600	1.400	1.200	1.000
Log of the ratio						
(lod score)	0.301	0.255	0.204	0.146	0.079	0.000

Table 6.2   Calculation of lod score for family B in Figure 6.1, given that the child is recombinant

	Linked					Unlinked
$\theta = 0.0$	0.1	0.2	0.3	0.4	0.5
Assuming loci are linked	0.000	0.100	0.200	0.300	0.400	0.500
Assuming loci are unlinked						0.500
Ratio linked : unlinked	0.000	0.200	0.400	0.600	0.800	1.000
Log of the ratio						
(lod score)	$-\infty$	-0.699	-0.398	-0.222	-0.097	0.000

Table 6.3   Calculation of lod score for family C in Figure 6.1, given that there are two nonrecombinant children

	Linked					Unlinked
$\theta = 0.0$	0.1	0.2	0.3	0.4	0.5
Linked	1.000	0.900	0.800	0.700	0.600	0.500
Linked	1.000	0.900	0.800	0.700	0.600	0.500
Total linked	1.000	0.810	0.640	0.490	0.360	0.250
Unlinked (child 1)						0.500
Unlinked (child 2)						0.500
Total unlinked						0.250
Ratio linked : unlinked	4.000	3.240	2.560	1.960	1.440	1.000
lod score	0.602	0.511	0.408	0.292	0.158	0.000

Table 6.4   Calculation of lod score for family D in Figure 6.1, given that there are five nonrecombinant children

		Linked				Unlinked
	θ = 0.0	0.1	0.2	0.3	0.4	0.5
If Linked						
Child 1	1.000	0.900	0.800	0.700	0.600	0.500
Child 2	1.000	0.900	0.800	0.700	0.600	0.500
Child 3	1.000	0.900	0.800	0.700	0.600	0.500
Child 4	1.000	0.900	0.800	0.700	0.600	0.500
Child 5	1.000	0.900	0.800	0.700	0.600	0.500
Total	1.000	0.590	0.328	0.168	0.078	0.031
If Unlinked						
Child 1						0.500
Child 2						0.500
Child 3						0.500
Child 4						0.500
Child 5						0.500
Total						0.031
Ratio linked : unlinked	32.00	18.90	10.49	5.378	2.488	1.000
lod score	1.505	1.276	1.021	0.731	0.396	0.000

Note: To conserve space or for simplicity of presentation, rounded numbers may be shown during the calculation. However, the unrounded, original numbers were used to calculate the final answer.

(14% recombination between the dominant disease locus and the DNA marker locus tested).

Instead of writing out a complex table of numbers to be multiplied, a formula provides the answer more quickly. For N total children, of whom R are recombinant and NR are nonrecombinant:

$$Z(\theta) = N(\log 2) + NR[\log(1 - \theta)] + R[\log \theta] \qquad (6.1)$$

or,

$$Z(\theta) = N(\log 2) \text{ when } \theta = 0 \qquad (6.2)$$

As an example, if a phase-known parent has ten children, comprising one recombinant and nine nonrecombinant

$$Z(\theta) = 10 (\log 2) + 9 [\log(1 - \theta)] + 1[\log \theta]$$

Table 6.5 Calculation of lod score for family E in Figure 6.1, given that the third of five children is recombinant

	Linked					Unlinked
θ = 0.0	0.1	0.2	0.3	0.4	0.5
			If Linked			
Child 1	1.000	0.900	0.800	0.700	0.600	0.500
Child 2	1.000	0.900	0.800	0.700	0.600	0.500
Child 3	0.000	0.100	0.200	0.300	0.400	0.500
Child 4	1.000	0.900	0.800	0.700	0.600	0.500
Child 5	1.000	0.900	0.800	0.700	0.600	0.500
Total	0.000	0.066	0.082	0.072	0.052	0.031
			If Unlinked			
Child 1						0.500
Child 2						0.500
Child 3						0.500
Child 4						0.500
Child 5						0.500
Total						0.031
Ratio linked : unlinked	0.000	2.100	2.621	2.305	1.659	1.000
lod score	$-\infty$	0.322	0.418	0.363	0.220	0.000

Note: To conserve space or for simplicity of presentation, rounded numbers may be shown during the calculation. However, the unrounded, original numbers were used to calculate the final answer.

Table 6.6 Cumulative lod score for all 5 families in Figure 6.1

		Linked					Unlinked
	θ = 0.0	0.1	0.2	0.3	0.4	0.5
Family A	1 NR : 0 R	0.301	0.255	0.204	0.146	0.079	0.000
Family B	0 NR : 1 R	$-\infty$	-0.699	-0.398	-0.222	-0.097	0.000
Family C	2 NR : 0 R	0.602	0.511	0.408	0.292	0.158	0.000
Family D	5 NR : 0 R	1.505	1.276	1.021	0.731	0.396	0.000
Family E	4 NR : 1 R	$-\infty$	0.322	0.418	0.363	0.220	0.000
Total	12 NR : 2 R	$-\infty$	1.665	1.653	1.310	0.756	0.000

If we substitute in $\theta = 0.1$ or $\theta = 0.25$, we get

$$Z(0.1) = 10 \, (\log 2) + 9[\log(0.9)] + 1[\log(0.1)]$$

which becomes

$$Z(0.1) = 10 \, (0.3010) + 9[-0.046] + 1[-1.000] = 1.598$$

which means that when $\theta = 0.1$ the lod score (Z) is 1.598, and

$$Z(0.25) = 10 \, (0.3010) + 9[\log(0.75)] + 1[\log(0.25)]$$
$$Z(0.25) = 3.010 + 9[-0.125] + 1[-0.602] = 1.284$$

which means that when $\theta = 0.25$, the lod score (Z) is 1.284.

Note that the two Z values above are not indicated as $\hat{Z}$ because we do not know this until we have determined Z at enough values of θ to establish where the maximum value occurs. Actually, of course, common sense tells us that the value at $\theta = 0.1$ will turn out to be the maximum $(\hat{\theta})$ because, in our head count, 1 out of 10 children was recombinant, giving a recombination fraction of 0.1.

The formula given above works only for phase-known meioses. For phase-unknown meioses, there is a further step to consider. If a father of unknown phase has five children, four with equivalent genotypic combinations inherited from him and one with a different genotypic combination inherited from him, two possibilities have to be considered: either his children represent 4NR:1R or they represent 1NR:4R, depending upon his (unknown) phase. This introduces ambiguity into the calculation and intuitively we should expect to obtain lower lod scores as a result of this uncertainty. In phase known meioses, the linked alleles are known to be in coupling, and the formula given above takes only this possibility into account. In the calculation for phase-unknown meioses, there is the additional possibility that the alleles were in repulsion and that the majority of the children are recombinant. We must therefore introduce a term into the formula to allow for this possibility.

For ten children with either two recombinant and eight nonrecombinant (8NR:2R) or eight recombinant and two nonrecombinant (2NR:8R), since we cannot tell the difference, these are entered as eight type A and two type B in the formula below.

$$Z(\theta) = N \, (\log 2) + \log\{[\theta^B * (1 - \theta)^A + (1 - \theta)^B * \theta^A]/2\}$$
$$Z(0.1) = 10 \, (\log 2) + \log\{[(0.1)^2 * (0.9)^8 + (0.9)^2 * (0.1)^8]/2\}$$
$$= 10 \, (0.301) + \log\{[0.01 * 0.430 + 0.81 * 1.0 * 10^{-8}]/2\}$$
$$= 3.010 + \log\{[0.0043 + 0.81 * 10^{-8}]/2\}$$
$$= 3.010 + \log\{0.00215\}$$
$$= 3.010 + (-2.667)$$
$$= 0.343$$

The single most important thing to remember about lod scores and maximum likelihood estimates of θ is that they are *estimates*. They are the best estimates with the data available to date. However, the first obligatory recombination event will send a huge positive lod score at $\hat{\theta} = 0.00$ crashing down to $-\infty$. It is because of the question, What impact will it have if the next child is recombinant? that methods of obtaining (estimating!) confidence intervals for estimates of θ have been devised.

Although there are many ways to determine confidence intervals for estimates of θ, one particular method was adopted as the standard method at the eighth human gene mapping conference in 1985 (Conneally et al. 1985). In this method, the lod scores obtained for a series of values of θ are plotted against θ on a graph. There will naturally be a peak somewhere on this graph, and we already know that this will represent $\hat{\theta}$ or our current best estimate of θ. The lod score at this value of θ is $\hat{Z}$. The confidence intervals are obtained by subtracting 1 from the value of $\hat{Z}$ and determining the values of θ where this lesser value of Z intersects the curve (if $\hat{\theta}$ was at 0, there will be only one additional value). If $\hat{Z}$ was 10.0 at $\hat{\theta} = 0.08$ and $\hat{Z} - 1$ intersects the curve at $\theta = 0.05$ and $\theta = 0.14$, then the best estimate of θ is stated to be 0.08 with a confidence interval (0.05–0.14). For small sample sizes (low values of $\hat{Z}$), the true value of $\hat{\theta}$ (as opposed to our estimate of it) will fall within the confidence interval at least 90% of the time; for larger sample sizes (high values of $\hat{Z}$), $\hat{\theta}$ will fall within the interval 95% of the time. The value of considering confidence intervals should be evident from considering what will happen to our estimate of $\hat{\theta}$ if the next meiosis happens to be recombinant (Table 6.7).

In each case, $\hat{Z}$ has decreased a little, and although the absolute value of $\hat{\theta}$ has almost doubled (as it should going from 1 recombinant out of N meioses to 2 recombinants out of N + 1), it is still well within the confidence interval of our estimate. The smaller the original number of recombination events, the greater the influence if the next meiosis happens to be recombinant. If the proportion of recombinants has always been high (e.g., 30 out of 100 meioses), it would not be a big surprise if the next meiosis included a recombination event, and this is reflected in the much smaller effect upon the estimates of $\hat{\theta}$ and $\hat{Z}$.

	$\hat{Z}$	$\hat{\theta}$	confidence interval
30/100 =	3.573	0.300	(0.208–0.403)
31/101 =	3.356	0.307	(0.215–0.410)

You will have already noticed that when we see values for $\hat{Z}$ and $\hat{\theta}$, it is not immediately obvious, from this information alone, how many

Table 6.7   Values of $\hat{Z}$, $\hat{\theta}$, and confidence intervals for
different numbers of recombinants and total phase-known
meioses

R/Tot	$\hat{Z}$	$\hat{\theta}$	Confidence Interval
1/200	57.47	0.005	(0.001–0.024)
2/201	55.64	0.010	(0.002–0.033)
1/100	27.67	0.010	(0.001–0.047)
2/101	26.14	0.020	(0.002–0.065)
1/50	12.92	0.020	(0.001–0.094)
2/51	11.69	0.039	(0.005–0.125)
1/20	4.30	0.050	(0.001–0.221)
2/21	3.45	0.095	(0.013–0.286)
1/15	2.92	0.067	(0.002–0.286)
2/16	2.20	0.125	(0.017–0.362)

Note: R/Tot = number of recombinant meioses/total number of
meioses.

meioses were studied and how many recombination events were noted.
Unfortunately, quite a few papers report maximum estimates for linkage data without confidence intervals. Perhaps you are considering performing tests for a condition that has been reported by independent groups, and having pooled their linkage data, you are wondering how much confidence to place in the new values of $\hat{Z}$ and $\hat{\theta}$. Situations such as these prompted me to find a way to "decode" lod scores so that an estimate would be available of just how much work is represented by $\hat{Z} = 3.0$ at $\hat{\theta} = 0.00$ or $\hat{Z} = 3.0$ at $\hat{\theta} = 0.40$. Try using the program discussed below on these numbers (0/10 and 137/343—there is a very large difference in the number of cases studied and therefore in the confidence intervals, +0.206 versus ±0.056).

Below is a sample output from a program written several years ago (in BASIC) to decode lod scores; the full listing of the program is given in the Appendix. (I apologize for the obvious lack of programing skill, but it works, and the logic is easier to follow when given one step at a time.) The algorithm that it uses to solve what appears to be one equation with two variables ($\hat{Z}$ and $\hat{\theta}$) works by initially comparing the entered $\hat{Z}$ to the $\hat{Z}$ that would be obtained if there were $100 * \hat{\theta}$ recombinants out of 100 phase-known meioses (converting recombination fraction literally to percentage recombinants). Comparison of this answer to the original value of $\hat{Z}$ gives the required ratio needed to obtain a very close approximation. Next it takes these numbers for recombinants and total meioses and recursively calculates the lod score from $\theta = 0.001$ up to $\hat{\theta}$ and from $\hat{\theta}$ up to 0.499 until it obtains values that equal $\hat{Z} - 1$. It reports these as the *approximate* confidence intervals. Finally, since the estimates are rarely integral numbers of people, it gives a selection of "whole" people around the estimate for you to choose from. As an example, 4.6 recombinants out of 23.2 phase-known meioses would be presented as $4/22$, $4/23$, $4/24$, $4/25$, $5/22$, etc., up to $6/25$. The initial estimates are nonintegral numbers because almost all linkage data contain some results derived from phase-unknown meioses. Since this program calculates how many phase-known meioses would be required, it always gives a minimum estimate of the actual work performed. It was only ever intended to give a crude guide.

```
ENTER THE VALUE OF Zmax TO BE DECODED
? 10.00
ENTER THE θmax FOR THAT VALUE OF Zmax
? .05
```

```
FIRST ESTIMATE IS 2.327575 RECOMBINANTS OUT OF    46.5515
PHASE-KNOWN MEIOSES WOULD GIVE Zmax = 10 AT θmax    = .05
CONFIDENCE INTERVALS FOR θ WOULD BE APPROXIMATELY .008 TO .148
RANGE OF INTEGRAL NUMBERS AROUND ESTIMATE—   TAKE YOUR PICK
```

RECOMBINANTS	MEIOSES	Zmax	θmax
1	45	11.4637	.0222222
1	46	11.75508	.0217391
1	47	12.04667	.0212766
1	48	12.33846	.0208333
2	45	9.992988	.0444444
2	46	10.2745	.0434783
2	47	10.55643	.0425532
2	48	10.83878	.0416667
3	45	8.759618	.0666667
3	46	9.031023	.0652174
3	47	9.303089	.0638298
3	48	9.575784	.0625

```
ENTER 1 TO CONTINUE, 2 TO QUIT OR 3 TO EXIT TO DOS
?
```

Since the numbers entered into the program were fictitious, it initially gives fractional numbers of people and meioses, shows approximate confidence intervals, and then leaves it to you to review the table of lod scores generated from an appropriate selection of integral numbers. In this particular case, 2 recombinants out of 45 phase-known informative meioses was about as close as we could get to the fictitious input.

I am indebted to an anonymous reviewer of the draft of this manuscript for pointing out to me that there is a published method to determine the "number of equivalent observations" that is similar to the core of the computer program (but does not give either approximate confidence intervals or a table of $\hat{Z}$ and $\hat{\theta}$ values for integral numbers). This method was described by Edwards (1976) and is also discussed in section 4.5 of the 1991 revised edition of Ott's book *Analysis of Human Genetic Linkage*. Starting with

$$Z(\theta) = N(\log 2) + NR[\log(1 - \theta)] + R[\log\theta] \tag{6.1}$$

we can take advantage of the fact that there is a special case when Z = $\hat{Z}$. When this is so, the best estimate of the recombination fraction is the number of recombinants over the total number of meioses, or $\hat{\theta}$ = R/N. The number of recombinants and nonrecombinants can then be determined by $R = \hat{\theta}N$ and $NR = (1 - \hat{\theta})N$. If we substitute for the unknown NR and R in equation 6.1, we get

$$\hat{Z} = N[\log(2) + (1 - \hat{\theta})\log(1 - \hat{\theta}) + (\hat{\theta})\log(\hat{\theta})] \tag{6.3}$$

or

$$\hat{Z} = N[\log(2)] \text{ when } \hat{\theta} = 0 \tag{6.4}$$

These rearrange to yield

$$N = \dot{Z}/[\log(2) + (1 - \dot{\theta})\log(1 - \dot{\theta}) + (\dot{\theta})\log(\dot{\theta})] \tag{6.5}$$

or

$$N = \hat{Z}/\log(2) \text{ when } \hat{\theta} = 0 \tag{6.6}$$

The number of recombinants, R, can be determined by

$$R = N\hat{\theta} \tag{6.7}$$

Thus, to use the same example as the computer program, if $\hat{Z}$ = 10.00 and $\hat{\theta}$ = 0.05,

$$
\begin{aligned}
N &= 10/[\log(2) + 0.95 * \log(0.95) + 0.05 * \log(0.05)] \\
&= 10/[0.301 + 0.95(-0.02228) + 0.05(-1.301)] \\
&= 10/[0.301 - 0.02116 - 0.06505] \\
&= 10/[0.2148] \\
&= 46.55.
\end{aligned}
$$

$R = 46.55 * 0.05 = 2.328$ (2.328 recombination events/46.55 meioses). As in the computer program, these numbers are nonintegral because the values for $\hat{Z}$ and $\hat{\theta}$ were ficticious.

Although the linkage approach can only give an estimate of the probability that the next meiosis will be recombinant, the estimate does represent the best interpretation of the data currently available. It is probably an error to build in further "margins of safety" by deliberately overestimating the probability of recombination in a diagnostic setting unless the value of $\hat{Z}$ is low. It is very tempting to do this, but if real laboratory results indicate that marker locus M recombines with disease locus D in 1% of meioses and the lod score is high, why pull a number such as 5% out of a hat "to be on the safe side"? That is not a scientific approach. Errors in the assumed value of $\hat{\theta}$ become quite serious when the probability of recombination is combined with other data such as biochemical test results or modification for incomplete penetrance or delayed onset. In section 8.2, a graph in Figure 8.5 shows the potentially disastrous effect of "adding a safety factor" to the recombination rate when considering age-at-onset corrections for a disease such as Huntington disease.

In the examples that we have studied, it has been assumed that the frequency of recombination is the same in males and in females. This was an approximation, since it is known that the rates are actually quite different and that, in general, the frequency of recombination is higher in females. To allow for this difference, the computer programs used to calculate lod scores have the capacity to study male and female meioses separately and to calculate θ_m and θ_f values instead of the average value that we have assumed. If this has been done, the appropriate sex-specific recombination rate can be used in risk calculations depending upon whether the disease may be passed through the mother or the father.

If we consider a polymorphic locus in band Xq28, at the bottom of the X chromosome, and measure the frequency with which recombination is observed between it and other loci further up the chromosome, we will initially detect perhaps 5% recombination with the nearby loci, then 10%, and then 20%. As we move progressively closer to the centromere, we will eventually reach a region that recombines with Xq28 in 50% of meioses (about band Xq25). This is only a fraction of the way up the chromosome, however, and every locus on the remaining 80–85% of the chromosome will also exhibit 50% recombination. Given that some of these loci are farther away than others, how do we determine their genetic distance from Xq28 or their order on the chromosome?

Throughout the last few pages, the discussion of recombinant and nonrecombinant offspring has assumed that they were the result of meioses with 1 or 0 crossover events, respectively. Actually, any even number of crossover events (counting zero as even) will generate offspring scored as nonrecombinant, and any odd number of crossover events will generate offspring scored as recombinant. Counting recombinant and nonrecombinant offspring therefore underestimates the frequency of crossover events, particularly for values of θ above 0.20. The observation of 50% recombination can therefore be the result of (*a*) independent assortment of different chromosomes (the loci are not syntenic and crossing over is irrelevant) or (*b*) any situation in which the loci are syntenic but unlinked because the frequency of an odd number of crossover events equals the frequency of an even number of crossover events. The maximum frequency of observed recombination is 50%; however, the probability of crossover events occurring between syntenic loci at opposite ends of one of the larger chromosomes may approach, or actually be, 100%.

To allow for the discrepancy between the observed rate of recombination and the number of crossover events, methods have been devised to convert percentage recombination or recombination fractions into map units. The unit of measurement in genetic maps is the centi-Morgan (cM). Loci may be more than 50 cM apart (the genetic map of the human X chromosome is slightly over 200 cM in length). There are several ways to convert recombination data into genetic maps, and the reader is referred to Ott (1991) for an authoritative discussion of these methods. For the purposes of the rest of this book, molecular diagnosis usually involves testing loci that have a low recombination fraction (0.10 or less) with the disease-causing locus, and under these special circumstances, recombination fractions, the probability of crossover events, and centiMorgans are approximately equal.

6.2   Probabilities over Pedigrees

The alternative method of calculating lod scores is to determine the mathematical probability of the whole pedigree occurring as stated, given particular values for allele frequencies and recombination fractions (probability over pedigree). This is a particularly useful approach, since computers can be programed to devise the specific equation for each family and can then proceed through an iterative process where they compare the total probability for each of a series of values of θ. The ratios of these probabilities can again be converted into lod scores, as in section 6.1.

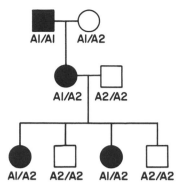

Figure 6.2 A family with a fully penetrant autosomal dominant disease that has been studied with a marker that has two alleles, A1 and A2. The cumulative probability of all of the genotypes within this family group (probability of the pedigree) is calculated in Table 6.8.

Assume that the family shown in Figure 6.2 has an autosomal dominant condition. The frequencies of alleles at the disease locus are d = 0.9999 and D = 0.0001, and the frequency of alleles at the marker locus are A1 = 0.6 and A2 = 0.4. Each person has two copies of that chromosome, and each chromosome has one copy of each locus. Four numbers can therefore be used to determine the total probability of each person's genotype (one number for each of the four positions). When the genotype of a person's parents is unknown, we use the Hardy-Weinberg equilibrium to obtain the population frequency of heterozygotes ($2pq$) or homozygotes (p^2 or q^2) at each locus. When the genotype of the parent is known, the probability of inheriting a particular allele is 1.0 from a homozygous parent or 0.5 from a heterozygous parent. For linkage calculations, once an allele at one of the loci (in this case the disease locus) has been determined, the probability of inheriting the allele at the second locus that was coupled to it in a phase-known meiosis is $1 - \theta$ (nonrecombinant offspring), and the probability of inheriting the allele that was originally in repulsion is θ (recombinant offspring).

Table 6.8 shows the derivation of the probability over a small, three-generation pedigree. In words, the probability for the genotype of I-1 is the probability that he is a heterozygote at the disease locus, ($2pq$) = (2 * 0.0001 * 0.9999), multiplied by the probability of being homozygous A1 at the marker locus (0.6 * 0.6). For III-1, it is the probability of inheriting the disease from her affected mother (0.5), multiplied by the probability of inheriting a normal allele from her father (1.0), multiplied by the probability of inheriting marker A1 from her phase-known mother, given that we already know that she has inherited the

Table 6.8   Probability of the pedigree shown in Figure 6.2

I-1	$2(0.0001 * 0.9999) * 0.6 * 0.6$	$= 7.2 * 10^{-5}$
I-2	$0.9999 * 0.9999 * 2(0.6 * 0.4)$	$= 0.48$
II-1	$0.5 * 1.0 * 1.0 * 0.5$	$= 0.25$
II-2	$0.9999 * 0.9999 * 0.4 * 0.4$	$= 0.16$
III-1	$0.5 * 1.0 * (1 - \theta) * 1.0$	$= 0.5(1 - \theta)$
III-2	$0.5 * 1.0 * (1 - \theta) * 1.0$	$= 0.5(1 - \theta)$
III-3	$0.5 * 1.0 * (1 - \theta) * 1.0$	$= 0.5(1 - \theta)$
III-4	$0.5 * 1.0 * (1 - \theta) * 1.0$	$= 0.5(1 - \theta)$

Cumulative probability of total pedigree $= 8.64 * 10^{-8}(1 - \theta)^4$

disease allele $(1 - \theta)$, multiplied by the probability of inheriting marker allele A2 from her father (1.0). Similar reasoning for the whole family leads to an expression for the cumulative probability of the total pedigree (Table 6.8).

When $\theta = 0.00$, this becomes $8.64 * 10^{-8} * (1.00)^4 = 8.64 * 10^{-8}$
When $\theta = 0.01$, this becomes $8.64 * 10^{-8} * (0.99)^4 = 8.30 * 10^{-8}$
When $\theta = 0.02$, this becomes $8.64 * 10^{-8} * (0.98)^4 = 7.97 * 10^{-8}$
When $\theta = 0.50$, this becomes $8.64 * 10^{-8} * (0.50)^4 = 5.40 * 10^{-9}$

These are directly convertible to lod scores by the relationship $Z(\theta)$ = the log of (Probability for any value of θ) divided by (Probability when $\theta = 0.50$)

$Z(0.00) = \log(8.64 * 10^{-8}/5.40 * 10^{-9}) = \log(16.00) = 1.20$
$Z(0.02) = \log(7.97 * 10^{-8}/5.40 * 10^{-9}) = \log(14.76) = 1.17$

The other appeal of this method is that it can be used for risk calculations merely by changing the parameter varied. If θ is kept constant at a given value, and the probability over the pedigree is calculated for two different genotypes of the consultand, two numbers can be derived: (a) the probability over the pedigree given that the consultand has the mutation and (b) the probability over the pedigree given that the consultand does not have the mutation. The ratio of these two numbers is obviously a direct estimate of genetic risk.

In the same pedigree, if we want to calculate the probability that III-4 has the mutation (as in, for example, a prenatal diagnosis), we just rearrange the logic a little so that θ is a known value, the marker locus is treated as the known factor, and the genotype of III-4 at the disease locus is the variable (Table 6.9).

Two lines are given for III-4: in the first calculation he is unaffected; in the second, affected. Put into words, the first line gives the probabil-

Table 6.9 Calculation of the probabilities of the pedigree in Figure 6.2 with 2 alternative genotypes for III-4 (e.g., affected or normal, as in a prenatal diagnosis)

I-1	$2(0.0001 * 0.9999) * 0.6 * 0.6$	$= 7.2 * 10^{-5}$
I-2	$0.9999 * 0.9999 * 2(0.6 * 0.4)$	$= 0.48$
II-1	$0.5 * 1.0 * 1.0 * 0.5$	$= 0.25$
II-2	$0.9999 * 0.9999 * 0.4 * 0.4$	$= 0.16$
III-1	$(1 - \theta) * 1.0 * 0.5 * 1.0$	$= 0.5(1 - \theta)$
III-2	$(1 - \theta) * 1.0 * 0.5 * 1.0$	$= 0.5(1 - \theta)$
III-3	$(1 - \theta) * 1.0 * 0.5 * 1.0$	$= 0.5(1 - \theta)$
III-4	$(1 - \theta) * 1.0 * 0.5 * 1.0$	$= 0.5(1 - \theta)$ Normal
III-4	$(\theta) * 1.0 * 0.5 * 1.0$	$= 0.5(\theta)$ Mutant

Cumulative probability when III-4 is normal $= 8.64 * 10^{-8} * (1 - \theta)^4$
Cumulative probability when III-4 is mutant $= 8.64 * 10^{-8} * \theta(1 - \theta)^3$

ity that III-4 inherited the normal allele at the disease locus given that we know that he inherited a maternal A2 allele at the marker locus $(1 - \theta)$ multiplied by the probabilities of inheriting a normal paternal allele (1.0), a maternal A2 allele (0.5), and a paternal A2 allele (1.0). The second line is the same except for the first term, which represents the probability of inheriting a mutant allele at the disease locus given that he inherited a maternal A2 allele at the marker locus (θ).

Let us assume that θ is known to be 0.02 and calculate his risk of possessing the mutant allele.

Probability if he is normal $= 8.64 * 10^{-8} * (0.98)^4 = 7.97 * 10^{-8}$
Probability if he is mutant $= 8.64 * 10^{-8} * (0.98)^3 * 0.02 = 1.63 * 10^{-9}$
Risk $=$ mutant/(mutant $+$ normal) $= 1.63/(79.7 + 1.63) = 0.020$

This answer is intuitively correct, since III-4 is the result of a phase-known meiosis when $\theta = 0.02$, and he inherited the A2 allele that was in coupling with the normal allele at the disease locus.

In the examples so far, the genotype of each person at the disease locus has been unambiguous. The approach gets a little more tedious to write out if several people are phase-unknown or if several people might or might not be carriers. In Figure 6.3, obligate carrier I-2 is phase-unknown and we do not know whether or not II-3 is a carrier, but want to calculate her risk. The following analysis was originally performed on a spreadsheet, writing out permutations of genotypes as columns and the probability of each event or dependent person's genotype as rows. Let us assume that alleles A1 and A2 occur with a frequency of 0.5 each and that the frequency of the disease allele (d) is 0.0001 (therefore $N = 0.9999$). This is presented in the format of a

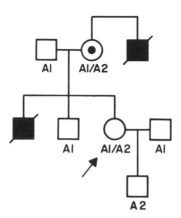

Figure 6.3   A phase-unknown family with an X-linked recessive disease. The daughter, II-3, is a potential carrier of the disease. In Table 6.10, the probability of this pedigree is calculated under four different assumptions: that she is either a carrier or a noncarrier for either potential phase in her mother. Her carrier risk can be determined from the ratio of these probabilities.

risk calculation (Table 6.10) using a value of $\theta = 0.10$, rather than a linkage calculation where θ is the unknown variable (θ would be substituted every time 0.1 appears below, and $1 - \theta$ every time 0.9 appears then, as earlier, a lod score could be obtained by comparing the probability of the pedigree for any given value of θ to that obtained when $\theta = 0.5$).

As already stated many times, the purpose of this book is not to be mathematically perfect to the sixth decimal place but to illustrate in a general sense the theory and methods used to calculate genetic risks. There is no intention to avoid the use of computer programs in risk calculation, but rather to ensure that their users are able to assess whether the answer obtained is approximately correct, so that the users can be confident that no serious error was made in data entry or in the genetic assumptions about the family.

This process can also be modified easily to accommodate the possibility of new mutations occurring in each gamete. The probability of inheriting a mutant gamete from an affected or carrier heterozygote is $0.5 + \mu$; the probability of inheriting a normal gamete from an affected or carrier heterozygote is $0.5 - \mu$; the probability of inheriting a normal gamete from a homozygous normal parent is $1 - \mu$; and the probability of inheriting a mutant gamete from a homozygous normal parent is μ. Note, however, that this assumes that mutations happen only in gametes, that is, the mutational event takes place following potential meiotic recombination, so terms involving θ are not combined with

Table 6.10 Calculation of carrier risk for II-3 in Figure 6.3 by comparing the probability of the whole pedigree with alternative states for her

		Phase in I-2			
		A1-N/A2-d		A1-d/A2-N	
	Status of II-3 =	Carrier	Noncarrier	Carrier	Noncarrier
		A1-N/A2-d	A1-N/A2-N	A1-N/A2-d	A1-N/A2-N
I-1	(A1-N)	$0.5 * 0.9999$	$0.5 * 0.9999$	$0.5 * 0.9999$	$0.5 * 0.9999$
I-2	(A1/A2,N/d)	$0.5 * 0.9999 * 0.5 * 0.0001$	$0.5 * 0.9999 * 0.5 * 0.0001$	$0.5 * 0.9999 * 0.5 * 0.0001$	$0.5 * 0.9999 * 0.5 * 0.0001$†
II-2	(A1-N)	$0.5 * 0.9$	$0.5 * 0.9$	$0.5 * 0.1$	$0.5 * 0.1$
II-3	(A1-N/A2-d)	$1 * 1 * 0.5 * 0.9$	$1 * 1 * 0.5 * 0.1$	$1 * 1 * 0.5 * 0.1$	
	(A1-N/A2-N)				$1 * 1 * 0.5 * 0.9$
II-4	(A1-N)	$0.5 * 0.9999$	$0.5 * 0.9999$	$0.5 * 0.9999$	$0.5 * 0.9999$
III-1	(A2-N)	$0.5 * 0.1$	$0.5 * 1$	$0.5 * 0.1$	$0.5 * 1$
Total		$6.3262 * 10^{-8}$	$7.0291 * 10^{-8}$	$7.8102 * 10^{-10}$	$7.0291 * 10^{-8}$

Carrier = columns $(1 + 3)/(1 + 2 + 3 + 4) = 6.4043 * 10^{-8}/2.0463 * 10^{-7} = 0.313$, or 31.3%

Note: The total probability of the pedigree when $\theta = 0.1$ (as calculated with the caveat indicated by the dagger) $= (1 + 2 + 3 + 4) = 2.046 * 10^{-7}$.

†This is actually a simplification, since I-2 obviously has a carrier mother; however, since we know nothing more about the mother, we used population frequencies for each component of her genotype. It makes no difference to the final outcome, since she has the same value in all columns. II-4 also makes no difference, since III-1 is male and does not inherit an X chromosome from his father.

terms involving μ [for example, the probability of inheriting a nonrecombinant mutant gamete from a heterozygous parent is considered to be $0.5(1 - \theta) + \mu$ and not $(0.5 + \mu)(1 - \theta)$]. Programers can obviously write their programs around whatever mutational theory they prefer. The one just mentioned is the simplest model to incorporate; however, as discussed earlier, meiotic mutations confined to a single gamete probably represent a minority of mutagenic events. If mutations are assumed to take place before meiosis (and recombination), the probability of inheriting a mutant gamete from an affected or carrier heterozygote is $(1 + \mu)/2$; the probability of inheriting a normal gamete from an affected or carrier heterozygote is $(1 - \mu)/2$; the probability of inheriting a normal gamete from a previously homozygous normal parent is $1 - \mu/2$; and the probability of inheriting a mutant gamete from a previously homozygous normal parent is $\mu/2$. Mathematical models can also go into sufficient depth to consider events such as back-mutations.

6.3   Multipoint Linkage Analysis

An important advance in methods of linkage analysis is called multipoint mapping. In the two-locus mapping described above, the hypothesis that the two loci are linked at a particular value of θ is compared with the hypothesis that the two loci are unlinked ($\theta = 0.5$), and the ratio between the likelihoods of each of these hypotheses is used to calculate a lod score. In multipoint mapping, the hypotheses are that the locus being tested falls within a specified interval containing two or more previously mapped loci or that it is far from (unlinked to) this interval. The results of this analysis are also in the form of an odds ratio, which is called a *location score*. Like lod scores, location scores are also logarithmic, but in natural logarithms (base e) rather than logarithms to the base 10. The location score would be calculated for a series of values as the test locus is moved across the interval under consideration. As an example, if we are testing whether a new polymorphic locus, C, falls within the interval between loci A and B, which are known to recombine in 2% of meioses ($\theta_{AB} = 0.02$), a series of calculations would be performed starting with locus C right next to locus A (e.g., $\theta_{AC} = 0.001$ and $\theta_{CB} = 0.019$) and slowly moving locus C across the interval until it is right next to locus B (e.g., $\theta_{AC} = 0.019$ and $\theta_{CB} = 0.001$). Each time, the probability (over the pedigree) of locus C being at that given position within the interval would be compared with the probability of its being unlinked. The location scores are given by $2 * \ln(\text{likelihood ratio})$, where the likelihood ratio

= (likelihood at the given position)/(likelihood unlinked to any marker within the interval), and a plot of these location scores against map distance will yield (for positive linkage) a graph with a series of peaks. The highest peak represents the most probable location of the new locus within the interval under investigation. Other possible locations are represented by the positions of smaller peaks. The probability that the new locus is at the most likely location rather than one of the alternatives is given by $e^{(X - Y)/2}$ where X and Y are the location scores of the two positions (e.g., if the most probable position, X, has a location score of 15 and the next most likely position, Y, a location score of 7, the odds that the new locus is at position X rather than Y are $e^{(15 - 7)/2} = e^4 = 55:1$). The other relevant feature on a graph of location scores is the presence of troughs, or valleys. These represent the positions of the loci that were already known to map within that interval (loci A and B in my description above).

Multipoint mapping is considered to be much more powerful than two-point mapping, and it will gain power as the linkage maps of the chromosomes become more densely saturated with DNA markers. The main drawbacks of this method are (*a*) that it is difficult to combine data from independent studies and (*b*) that the validity of the results are questionable unless the existing map of the control loci against which the new locus is being mapped is known to be very accurate.

Multipoint mapping is also particularly useful for exclusion of linkage from a given interval; for example, if the new locus is excluded from a fairly large interval such as locus P – ($\theta_{PQ} = 0.20$) – locus Q – ($\theta_{QR} = 0.15$) – locus R – ($\theta_{RS} = 0.25$) – locus S – ($\theta_{ST} = 0.20$) – locus T (for illustrative purposes only; an interval of this size would be mapped in cM rather than percentage recombination), it will have been excluded from a sizeable fraction of a chromosomal arm in a single analysis. A series of similar negative results will soon lead to very few remaining possibilities in the genome for the new locus. Exclusion mapping by this method is very much faster than by two-point analyses.

7

Use of DNA Markers
to Predict Genetic Risks

This chapter contains examples of the application of DNA markers to the prediction of genotype at a disease-causing locus that is inherited in an X-linked, an autosomal dominant, or an autosomal recessive mode. Each section starts with an easy example (usually a small phase-known pedigree) and then progresses to more difficult analyses (usually phase-unknown). Almost all of the pedigrees are small (a) because most pedigrees encountered by diagnostic laboratories actually are small (unlike the gigantic multigenerational pedigrees so often collected for gene mapping), (b) because it is easier to type out the relevant calculations, and (c) because, as we shall see, sometimes the smallest pedigrees are very difficult to analyze—the probability of phase usually increases in parallel with size of the pedigree.

7.1 Single Markers in Familial Cases

7.1.1 X-linked Inheritance

In their classic book, Murphy and Chase (1975, pp. 207–8) gave one example of a calculation that included linkage data in the estimation of genetic risk to a consultand. In their example, genotypes at the G6PD locus (although they actually omitted the genotypes of several key individuals) were used to help calculate the risk that the consultand was a carrier of hemophilia A. The known linkage at $\theta = 0.05$ was used as a conditional probability and generated a column ratio of $19:1$, which was considerably in excess of the ratios given for most of their

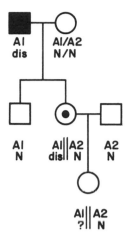

Figure 7.1   A phase-known family with positive family history of an X-linked recessive disease. Marker locus A is linked to the disease locus at θ = 0.02. The risk that III-1 is a carrier is calculated in Table 7.1.

Table 7.1   Determination of the carrier risk for III-1 in Figure 7.1 where her mother is phase-known

| Phase in II-2 | Al-dis/A2-N | |
| Probability of phase | 1.00 | |
III-1 =	Carrier	Noncarrier
Prior probability	0.5	0.5
Conditional probability		
maternal A1	0.98	0.02
Joint probability	0.49	0.01
Posterior probability	0.98	0.02

Bayesian calculations. This was also combined with biochemical test results (factor VIII assay) to obtain the overall risk.

In Figure 7.1, I-1 has hemophilia B and has two children. His daughter, II-2, is an obligate carrier and, after exhausting all of the intragenic markers, is found to be heterozygous only at locus A, which recombines with the disease locus in 2% of meioses. Because we have studied her affected father, who has marker allele A1 on his single X chromosome, her phase is known to be A1-dis/A2-N. She has passed on the same A1 allele to her daughter, III-1, who will therefore be a carrier of hemophilia B (98% probability) unless recombination took place during oogenesis (2% probability) (Table 7.1).

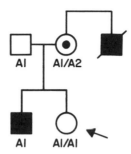

Figure 7.2   A phase-unknown family with a positive family history of an X-linked recessive disease. Marker locus A is linked to the disease locus at θ = 0.10. The risk that II-2 is a carrier is calculated in Table 7.2.

Table 7.2   Determination of the carrier risk for II-2 in Figure 7.2 where her mother is phase-unknown

| | Phase in I-2 | | | |
	A1-dis/A2-N		A1-N/A2-dis	
Prior probability	0.5		0.5	
Conditional probability				
son is A1-dis†	0.9		0.1	
Joint probability	0.45		0.05	
Posterior probability	0.9		0.1	
II-2 =	Carrier	Noncarrier	Carrier	Noncarrier
Conditional probability				
maternal A1	0.9	0.1	0.1	0.9
Joint probability	0.81	0.09	0.01	0.09

Carrier total = 0.81 + 0.01 = 0.82
Noncarrier total = 0.09 + 0.09 = 0.18

† The probability that a son who is affected would also have inherited allele A1 if the phase in the mother is as shown at the top of each column. This is taking a few short-cuts from the approach used in obtaining probabilities of pedigrees which would also take into account the probability of his being affected (0.5 ∗ 0.9 or 0.5 ∗ 0.1).

In Figure 7.2, I-2 is an obligate carrier who is heterozygous at marker locus A but phase-unknown. The recombination fraction is 0.10. Her most likely phase can be determined as A1-dis/A2-N by the fact that she passed allele A1 with the disease to her son (Table 7.2). II-2 is a carrier when (a) both she and her affected brother are nonrecombinant

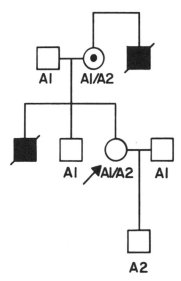

Figure 7.3 A phase-unknown family with a positive family history of an X-linked recessive disease. Marker locus A is linked to the disease locus at θ = 0.10. II-3 is a potential carrier. Her risk is calculated in Table 7.3 taking into account that she has a normal son who inherited the "at-risk" marker allele from a phase-known meiosis. She can be a carrier only if her son is recombinant.

(81%) and (*b*) both are recombinant (1%). She is a noncarrier when (*c*) she alone is recombinant (9%) or (*d*) he alone is recombinant (9%).

In Figure 7.3, II-3 is similarly the daughter of a heterozygous but phase-unknown obligate carrier. In this example, she inherited the maternal allele opposite to her normal brother's. As in the preceding example, if θ = 0.10, she has an 82% risk of being a carrier of the disease. If she is a carrier, she is also phase-known (A1-N/A2-dis), since we have studied her normal father. One additional piece of information is available with the presence of her normal son, who inherited the grandmaternal A2 allele (Table 7.3). The fact that she passed the "at-risk" DNA allele to her normal son has reduced her carrier risk from 82% to 31%; she can be a carrier only if her normal son is recombinant.

7.1.2 Autosomal Dominant Inheritance

Let us assume that prenatal diagnosis has been requested by the family in Figure 7.4 for a fully penetrant autosomal dominant condition. The recombination fraction between marker locus A and the dis-

Table 7.3   Calculation of carrier risk for II-3 in Figure 7.3 with inclusion of posterior information

	Carrier	Noncarrier
Phase in II-3 =	A1-N/A2-dis	A1-N/A2-N
Prior probability	0.82	0.18
Conditional probability		
A2-N son	0.10	1.00
Joint probability	0.082	0.18
Posterior probability	0.313	0.687

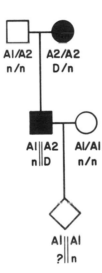

Figure 7.4   A phase-known family with a positive family history of a fully pene-trant autosomal dominant disease. Marker locus A is linked to the disease locus at θ = 0.01. Since the fetus III-1 inherited the grandpaternal A1 allele from a phase-known meiosis, it can be affected only if recombination took place.

ease is 0.01. Affected male II-1 is phase-known, since we know that he inherited both the disease and allele A2 from his affected mother. He passed the grandpaternal A1 allele to the fetus, which is therefore at low risk of having inherited the disease (1%).

In Figure 7.5, only two generations were available for analysis, so the pedigree is technically phase-unknown. The phase in the affected mother, I-2, can be inferred from the fact that she passed VNTR allele A3 to her normal son and allele A8 to her affected daughter. If θ =

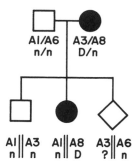

Figure 7.5   A phase-unknown family with a positive family history of a fully penetrant autosomal dominant disease. VNTR marker locus A is linked to the disease
locus at θ = 0.02. The probabilities of the potential phases in I-2 and the risk for
II-3 are calculated in Table 7.4.

Table 7.4   Calculation of the probability that the fetus, II-3, in Figure 7.5 will be
affected by the autosomal dominant disease

	Phase in I-2			
	A3-D/A8-n		A3-n/A8-D	
Prior probability	0.5		0.5	
Conditional probabilities				
II-1 A3-n	0.02		0.98	
II-2 A8-D	0.02		0.98	
Joint probability	0.0002		0.4802	
Posterior probability	0.0004		0.9996	
II-3 =	Affected	Normal	Affected	Normal
Conditional probability				
maternal A3	0.98	0.02	0.02	0.98
Joint probability	0.000392	0.000008	0.019992	0.979608

Total D (affected) = 0.000392 + 0.019992 = 0.020384 (2%)
Total n (normal)   = 0.000008 + 0.979608 = 0.979616 (98%)

0.02, the probabilities of the potential phases in I-2 can be calculated,
and then applied to II-3, as shown in Table 7.4.

7.1.3   Autosomal Recessive Inheritance

Phase-known pedigrees tend to be three-generation pedigrees where
the phase is proven in the second generation because it is known spe-

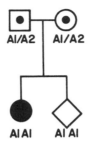

Figure 7.6   A family with an autosomal recessive disease. The parents are not believed to be consanguineous. Marker locus A is linked to the disease locus at θ
= 0.05. The probabilities of each potential phase in both parents are calculated
in Table 7.5 and then used to predict the likelihoods of potential genotypes
in II-2.

cifically which grandparent was the source of the disease-causing mutation. In the absence of consanguinity, it is extremely rare to have a
truly phase-known pedigree for an autosomal recessive disorder. In
DNA analysis for autosomal recessive disorders, therefore, the phase
in the parents is almost always inferred from their offspring. In a paper
on the estimation of error rates in diagnosis with linked markers, Kadasi (1989) pointed out that for autosomal recessive inheritance, recombination has four opportunities to interfere with the diagnostic
process: two in the determination of probable phase in both parents,
and two in the application of the likelihood of those phases to the
consultand.

In the family in Figure 7.6, the first child is affected with a rare
autosomal recessive condition, but there is no known consanguinity
between the parents. Marker locus A recombines with the disease in
5% of meioses. Since the affected child is homozygous A1/A1, the
obvious inference is that the disease is probably coupled to A1 in
both parents (95% posterior probability each). We can construct the
following table of combinations of genotypes; for each fetal genotype,
the two products for the father are added and then multiplied by the
equivalent sum for the mother. In Table 7.5, the first bracketed numbers on the line representing the total risk of being affected are derived
from (0.95 * 0.95 + 0.05 * 0.05), which is the probability that the phase
in the father is A1-d/A2-N (0.95), multiplied by the probability of the
meiotic event that would give the fetus a mutant allele (0.95), plus
the probability of the opposite phase in the father (0.05), multiplied
by the probability of the necessary meiotic event (0.05). This is then
multiplied by the value obtained from the numbers in the second
bracket, which represent the same components from the mother.

Table 7.5 Calculation of (i) the probable phase of each parent in Figure 7.6 based upon the genotype of their affected child, and (ii) the probable genotype of their next child

| | Potential Phase in | | | |
| | Father | | Mother | |
	A1-d/A2-N	A1-N/A2-d	A1-d/A2-N	A1-N/A2-d
Posterior probability based on II-1	0.95	0.05	0.95	0.05
	Probability that in II-2			
A1-pat/A1-mat = dd	0.95	0.05	0.95	0.05
= Nd	0.05	0.95	0.95	0.05
= dN	0.95	0.05	0.05	0.95
= NN	0.05	0.95	0.05	0.95

Total dd (affected) $= (0.9025 + 0.0025) * (0.9025 + 0.0025) = 0.819$
Total Nd (carrier) $= 2(0.0475 + 0.0475) * (0.9025 + 0.0025) = 0.172$
Total NN (noncarrier) $= (0.0475 + 0.0475) * (0.0475 + 0.0475) = 0.009$

II-2 therefore has an 82% probability of being affected, a 17% probability of being a carrier, and a 1% probability of being a noncarrier.

7.2 Flanking Markers in Familial Cases

7.2.1 X-linked Inheritance

In Figure 7.7, II-1 is phase-known A1-dis-B1/A2-N-B2. Since III-2 inherited the A2-B2 chromosome from her mother, she is a noncarrier unless a double crossover occurred. Single crossovers are ruled out by the fact that the haplotype on her maternal chromosome is not A1-B2 or A2-B1. If $\theta_A = \theta_B = 0.10$, then

Probability of no crossovers $= 0.9 * 0.9 = 0.81$
Probability of double crossover $= 0.1 * 0.1 = 0.01$
Carrier risk $= 0.01/(0.81 + 0.01) = 0.01/0.82 = 0.0122$, or 1.2%

In Figure 7.8, the mother, I-2, is phase-unknown, but she has two affected sons, and her phase can be inferred from their genotypes (modified from Bridge and Lillicrap 1989). The four possible phases in mother I-2 are

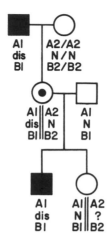

Figure 7.7   A phase-known family with a positive family history of an X-linked recessive disease. Marker loci A and B flank (are on opposite sides of) the disease locus, and both recombine with it at $\theta = 0.10$. The risk for III-2 is discussed in the text.

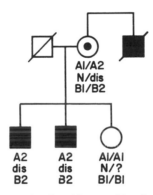

Figure 7.8   A phase-unknown family with a positive family history of an X-linked recessive disease. Marker loci A and B flank the disease locus at $\theta_A = 0.09$ and $\theta_B = 0.14$. There are four potential maternal phases to consider in pedigrees with phase-unknown flanking markers; the probabilities of each of these are calculated in Table 7.6, and the probability that II-3 is a carrier is calculated from these in Table 7.7.

C	D	E	F
A2-dis-B2	A1-dis-B2	A2-dis-B1	A1-dis-B1
A1-NOR-B1	A2-NOR-B1	A1-NOR-B2	A2-NOR-B2

The probability of having two affected sons with A2-dis-B2 genotypes for each possible maternal phase, assuming a recombination fre-

Table 7.6 Calculation of the probability of each of four potential maternal phases in Figure 7.8 based upon the genotypes of her two affected sons

Maternal Phase	Son II-1		Son II-2			Total	%
	A	B	A	B			
C	0.91 *	0.86 *	0.91 *	0.86 =		0.612463	96.5
D	0.09 *	0.86 *	0.09 *	0.86 =		0.005991	0.944
E	0.91 *	0.14 *	0.91 *	0.14 =		0.016231	2.56
F	0.09 *	0.14 *	0.09 *	0.14 =		0.000159	0.0250

Table 7.7 Determination of the carrier risk of II-3 in Figure 7.8 based upon the likelihood of each potential maternal phase

Maternal Phase	Probability of Phase	A		B		Total
		II-3 Carrier				
C	96.5	0.09 *		0.14 =		1.215581
D	0.944	0.91 *		0.14 =		0.120222
E	2.56	0.09 *		0.86 =		0.197885
F	0.0250	0.91 *		0.86 =		0.019571
Total = 1.553259 = 2% carrier						
		II-3 Noncarrier				
C	96.5	0.91 *		0.86 =		75.50108
D	0.94	0.09 *		0.86 =		0.073039
E	2.56	0.91 *		0.14 =		0.325718
F	0.025	0.09 *		0.14 =		0.000315
Total = 75.90015 = 98% noncarrier						

quency of 0.09 (9%) for θ_A and of 0.14 (14%) for θ_B, is shown in Table 7.6. These are the relative likelihoods of the possible phase arrangements in I-2, based upon her sons' genotypes. The probabilities that daughter II-3 is a carrier or a noncarrier are calculated from the probabilities of the maternal phases and the various recombination events necessary to make the daughter a carrier or a noncarrier starting from each maternal phase (Table 7.7).

The four possible phases for the mother, I-2, in Figure 7.9 are

	G	H	I	J
	A2-dis-B1	A2-dis-B1	A1-dis-B2	A2-dis-B2
	A2-NOR-B2	A1-NOR-B2	A2-NOR-B1	A1-NOR-B1

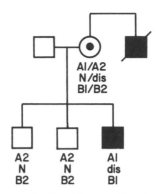

Figure 7.9   A phase-unknown family with a positive family history of an X-linked recessive disease. Marker loci A and B flank the disease locus at $\theta_A = 0.09$ and $\theta_B = 0.10$. Obligate carrier I-2 wants to have more children. The probabilities of all possible marker haplotypes for a future child, along with the genetic risk associated with each haplotype, are calculated in Tables 7.8 to 7.15.

Table 7.8   Calculation of the probability of each potential maternal phase in Figure 7.9

Maternal Phase	Son II-1		Son II-2		Son II-3		Total	%
	A	B	A	B	A	B		
G	0.91 *	0.90 *	0.91 *	0.90 *	0.91 *	0.90 =	0.549353	99.8
H	0.09 *	0.90 *	0.09 *	0.90 *	0.09 *	0.90 −	0.000531	0.0965
I	0.91 *	0.10 *	0.91 *	0.10 *	0.91 *	0.10 =	0.000754	0.137
J	0.09 *	0.10 *	0.09 *	0.10 *	0.09 *	0.10 =	0.000001	0.000132

Note: To conserve space or for simplicity of presentation, rounded numbers may be shown during the calculation. However, the unrounded, original numbers were used to calculate the final answer.

The probability of having two unaffected sons with A2-N-B2 genotypes and one affected son with an A1-dis-B1 genotype for each possible maternal phase, assuming a recombination frequency of 0.09 (9%) for θ_A and of 0.10 (10%) for θ_B, is shown in Table 7.8. These are the relative likelihoods of the possible phase arrangements in I-2 based upon her sons' genotypes.

For the sake of illustration, let us assume that I-2 wants to have more children, that the couple are very well educated and are asking very pointed questions about the accuracy with which you can test the next pregnancy. You satisfy them with the following in-depth analysis, which takes all possible fetal genotypes and, in turn, predicts the fre-

Table 7.9 Calculation of the risk associated with fetal genotype P (A2-?-B2)

Maternal Phase	Phase %		A		B		Total
		? = dis					
G	99.8	*	0.09	*	0.10	=	0.89790
H	0.0965	*	0.91	*	0.10	=	0.00878
I	0.137	*	0.09	*	0.90	=	0.01109
J	0.000132	*	0.91	*	0.90	=	0.00011
Total = 0.91787							
Risk = (1.11%)							
		? = N					
G	99.8	*	0.91	*	0.90	=	81.7088
H	0.0965	*	0.09	*	0.90	=	0.00782
I	0.137	*	0.91	*	0.10	=	0.01245
J	0.000132	*	0.09	*	0.10	=	0.00000
Total = 81.7290							
Risk = (98.89%)							

Note: To conserve space or for simplicity of presentation, rounded numbers may be shown during the calculation. However, the unrounded, original numbers were used to calculate the final answer.

quency with which each would be expected to occur as well as the risk associated with each marker haplotype.

The possible genotypes of a hypothetical male fetus in Figure 7.9 are

P	Q	R	S
A2-?-B2	A1-?-B2	A2-?-B1	A1-?-B1

Conditional risks will be calculated for ? = dis and ? = N in Tables 7.9 to 7.12 by combining the probabilities of the possible maternal phases with the likelihoods of the recombination events necessary to generate each genotype from the relevant maternal arrangement. Table 7.13 shows the summary of the risks determined in Tables 7.9 to 7.12. For each hypothetical fetal genotype, the posterior risk of ? = mutant or ? = normal is given.

The analysis of the possibilities for this family can be concluded by calculating the frequency with which each of these hypothetical male fetal genotypes might be expected to occur. The frequencies of the hypothetical male fetal genotypes, P, Q, R, and S, are derived from

Table 7.10   Calculation of the risk associated with fetal
genotype Q (A1-?-B2)

Maternal Phase	Phase %		A		B		Total
			? = dis				
G	99.8	*	0.91	*	0.10	=	9.07875
H	0.0965	*	0.09	*	0.10	=	0.00087
I	0.137	*	0.91	*	0.90	=	0.11208
J	0.000132	*	0.09	*	0.90	=	0.00001
Total = 9.19171							
Risk = (52.97%)							
			? = N				
G	99.8	*	0.09	*	0.90	=	8.08109
H	0.0965	*	0.91	*	0.90	=	0.07904
I	0.137	*	0.09	*	0.10	=	0.00123
J	0.000132	*	0.91	*	0.10	=	0.00001
Total = 8.16137							
Risk = (47.03%)							

Note: To conserve space or for simplicity of presentation,
rounded numbers may be shown during the calculation. However,
the unrounded, original numbers were used to calculate the final
answer.

the probabilities of each of the potential maternal phase arrangements
and the likelihoods of the number and type of recombination events
required to generate each fetal genotype from the relevant maternal
arrangement.

The frequency of various recombination events for any maternal
phase can be computed from the products of the relevant values of θ
(recombination did occur) or $1 - \theta$ (recombination did not occur).

Nonrecombinant	$0.90 * 0.91 = 0.8190$
Single recombinant A-dis	$0.90 * 0.09 = 0.0810$
Single recombinant B-dis	$0.10 * 0.91 = 0.0910$
Double recombinant A-dis-B	$0.10 * 0.09 = 0.0090$

For each maternal phase, each fetal genotype will occur as the result
of either (*a*) no crossover or a double crossover, or (*b*) a single crossover either above or below the disease locus (Table 7.14).

Frequency of (*a*) = 0.8190 + 0.0090 = 0.8280
Frequency of (*b*) = 0.0810 + 0.0910 = 0.1720

Table 7.11 Calculation of the risk associated with fetal genotype R (A2-?-B1)

Maternal Phase	Phase %		A		B		Total
		? = dis					
G	99.8	*	0.09	*	0.90	=	8.08109
H	0.0965	*	0.91	*	0.90	=	0.07904
I	0.137	*	0.09	*	0.10	=	0.00123
J	0.000132	*	0.91	*	0.10	=	0.00001
Total = 8.16137							
Risk = 47.03%							
		? = N					
G	99.8	*	0.91	*	0.10	=	9.07875
H	0.0965	*	0.09	*	0.10	=	0.00087
I	0.137	*	0.91	*	0.90	=	0.11208
J	0.000132	*	0.09	*	0.90	=	0.00001
Total = 9.19171							
Risk = 52.97%							

Note: To conserve space or for simplicity of presentation, rounded numbers may be shown during the calculation. However, the unrounded, original numbers were used to calculate the final answer.

Table 7.15 summarizes the series of calculations performed in Tables 7.9 to 7.14, giving the predicted frequency of each potential fetal genotype and the likelihood that each will be mutant or normal.

7.2.2 Autosomal Dominant Inheritance

In Figure 7.10, let us assume that prenatal diagnosis has been requested by II-1 for an autosomal dominant disease for which flanking markers are available; $\theta_A = 0.04$ and $\theta_B = 0.02$. Since II-1 is phase-known, the calculation proceeds in the same manner as the phase-known flanking marker calculation for an X-linked disease, as in Figure 7.7.

The fetus, III-2, has inherited the grandmaternal haplotype from the mother and will be affected unless a double crossover has taken place. Single crossover events have been excluded by the failure to find a recombinant maternal A1-B1 or A2-B2 haplotype in the fetus.

Table 7.12   Calculation of the risk associated with fetal
genotype S (A1-?-B1)

Maternal Phase	Phase %	A		B		Total
		? = dis				
G	99.8	* 0.91	*	0.90	=	81.7088
H	0.0965	* 0.09	*	0.90	=	0.00782
I	0.137	* 0.91	*	0.10	=	0.01245
J	0.000132	* 0.09	*	0.10	=	0.00000

   Total = 81.7290
   Risk = 98.89%

Maternal Phase	Phase %	A		B		Total
		? = N				
G	99.8	* 0.09	*	0.10	=	0.89790
H	0.0965	* 0.91	*	0.10	=	0.00878
I	0.137	* 0.09	*	0.90	=	0.01109
J	0.000132	* 0.91	*	0.90	=	0.00011

   Total = 0.91787
   Risk = 1.11%

Note: To conserve space or for simplicity of presentation,
rounded numbers may be shown during the calculation. However,
the unrounded, original numbers were used to calculate the final
answer.

Table 7.13   Summary of risks for each possible fetal genotype

	Hypothetical Fetal Genotype			
	P	Q	R	S
Posterior risk				
? = dis	1.11%	52.97%	47.03%	98.89%
? = N	98.89%	47.03%	52.97%	1.11%

Probability of no crossover   = 0.96 * 0.98   = 0.9408
Probability of double crossover   = 0.04 * 0.02   = 0.0008
Risk = 0.9408/(0.9408 + 0.0008) = 0.9408/0.9416 = 0.9992 = 99.9%

In Figure 7.11, I-2 is phase-unknown because we did not have an
opportunity to study her parents. The phase of the alleles at marker
loci A and B with respect to the disease-causing mutation can nevertheless be inferred from her two affected children; $\theta_A = 0.05$ and θ_B

Table 7.14   Predicted frequency of the four possible fetal
genotypes if I-2 in Figure 7.9 has another child

Maternal Phase	Phase %	Recombination†		Total
		Fetal Genotype P		
G	99.8	* 0.8280	=	82.6067
H	0.0965	* 0.1720	=	0.01660
I	0.137	* 0.1720	=	0.02354
J	0.000132	* 0.8280	=	0.00011
Total = 82.6469				
Risk = 41.3%				
		Fetal Genotype Q		
G	99.8	* 0.1720	=	17.1598
H	0.0965	* 0.8280	=	0.07991
I	0.137	* 0.8280	=	0.11332
J	0.000132	* 0.1720	=	0.00002
Total = 17.3531				
Risk = 8.7%				
		Fetal Genotype R		
G	99.8	* 0.1720	=	17.1598
H	0.0965	* 0.8280	=	0.07991
I	0.137	* 0.8280	=	0.11332
J	0.000132	* 0.1720	=	0.00002
Total = 17.3531				
Risk = 8.7%				
		Fetal Genotype S		
G	99.8	* 0.8280	=	82.6067
H	0.0965	* 0.1720	=	0.01660
I	0.137	* 0.1720	=	0.02354
J	0.000132	* 0.8280	=	0.00011
Total = 82.6469				
Risk = 41.3%				

Note: To conserve space or for simplicity of presentation, rounded numbers may be shown during the calculation. However, the unrounded, original numbers were used to calculate the final answer.

†This column represents the probability of either no crossover, a double crossover, or single crossovers.

Table 7.15   Summary of the risks for a future child in Figure 7.9

Potential Male Fetal Genotype	Predicted Frequency	Likelihood That ? = dis	Likelihood That ? = N
P A2-?-B2	41.3%	1.11%	98.89%
Q A1-?-B2	8.7%	52.97%	47.03%
R A2-?-B1	8.7%	47.03%	52.97%
S A1-?-B1	41.3%	98.89%	1.11%

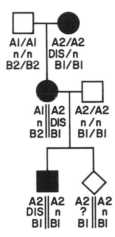

Figure 7.10   A phase-known family with a positive family history of a fully penetrant autosomal dominant disease. Marker loci A and B flank the disease locus at
$\theta_A = 0.04$ and $\theta_B = 0.02$. The fetus, III-2, has inherited the high-risk grandmaternal haplotype from its mother and will be affected unless it is a double recombinant.

= 0.03. The process is to calculate retrospectively the probability of
each possible maternal phase, based upon the fact that she already has
two affected children with specific genotypes. From each potential
maternal phase, we can then calculate the probability that the fetus
will be affected or will be normal, depending upon what crossover
events would be required to generate each state for its known A2-B1
maternal haplotype (Table 7.16). The fetus therefore has a 99.8%
chance of being normal and a 0.2% chance of being affected.

7.2.3   Autosomal Recessive Inheritance

In the case of autosomal recessive diseases, probably all pedigrees
except consanguineous ones will be phase-unknown. In Figure 7.12, a

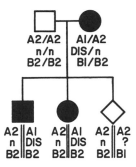

Figure 7.11   A phase-unknown family with a positive family history of a fully penetrant autosomal dominant disease. Marker loci A and B flank the disease locus
at $\theta_A = 0.05$ and $\theta_B = 0.03$. The probabilities of the four possible phases in I-2
and the risk that II-3 will be affected are calculated in Table 7.16.

Table 7.16   Possible phases in I-2 in Figure 7.11 (only disease-bearing
chromosome shown)

	A1-D-B1	A1-D-B2	A2-D-B1	A2-D-B2
Prior probability	0.25	0.25	0.25	0.25
II-1 A1-D	0.95	0.95	0.05	0.05
D-B2	0.03	0.97	0.03	0.97
II-2 A1-D	0.95	0.95	0.05	0.05
D-B2	0.03	0.97	0.03	0.97
Joint probability	0.000203063	0.212290563	0.000000563	0.000588063
Posterior probability	0.000952957	0.996260894	0.000002642	0.002759728
Risk that II-3 in Figure 7.11 is A2-D-B1				
A2-D	0.05	0.05	0.95	0.95
D-B1	0.97	0.03	0.97	0.03
Joint probability	0.000046218	0.001494391	0.000002435	0.000078652
Total for A2-D-B1 = 0.001621696				
Risk that II-3 in Figure 7.11 is A2-n-B1				
A2-n	0.95	0.95	0.05	0.05
n-B1	0.03	0.97	0.03	0.97
Joint probability	0.000027159	0.918054414	0.000000004	0.000133847
Total for A2-n-B1 = 0.918215424				

Risk normal = 0.918215424/(0.918215424 + 0.001621696) = 0.99824
Risk affected = 0.001621696/(0.918215424 + 0.001621696) = 0.00176

Note: To conserve space or for simplicity of presentation, rounded numbers may be
shown during the calculation. However, the unrounded, original numbers were used to
calculate the final answer.

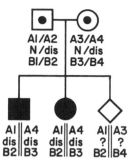

Figure 7.12   A family with an autosomal recessive disease. Marker loci A and B flank the disease locus at $\theta_A = 0.05$ and $\theta_B = 0.20$. The parents are not believed to be consanguineous. The probabilities of the four possible phases in each parent are calculated in Table 7.17 and the risks that II-3 is affected, a carrier, or a noncarrier are calculated from these in Table 7.18.

couple who already have two affected children elect to pursue DNA testing for their third pregnancy. Marker loci A and B flank the disease locus, and $\theta_A = 0.05$ and $\theta_B = 0.20$. For an autosomal recessive disease, we need to calculate the probability of four potential phases in each parent (Table 7.17) and then determine the probability of the fetus's possessing the mutation within the haplotypes inherited from both parents.

The two fetal haplotypes can have four states of affection A1-?-B2/A3-?-B4, where ?? = dd, dN, Nd, or NN, representing affected, carrier, carrier, and noncarrier, respectively. With the appropriate cross-over events, the fetus can have either d or N within both of its haplotypes, so the probability of each must be calculated from each potential maternal and paternal phase, and the sum of all these independent probabilities added together to obtain the final risks of being affected, a carrier, or a noncarrier.

The first line in the dd (affected) calculation in Table 7.18 represents (d from paternal phase A1-d-B1 plus d from paternal phase A1-d-B2 plus d from paternal phase A2-d-B1 plus d from paternal phase A2-d-B2) * (d from maternal phase A3-d-B3 plus d from maternal phase A3-d-B4 plus d from maternal phase A4-d-B3 plus d from maternal phase A4-d-B4). For the fetus with a paternal A1-?-B2, to inherit d from paternal phase A1-d-B1 (posterior probability 0.058661033) would require no crossover with the A locus (0.95) but would require a cross-over with the B locus (0.20) = 0.058661033 * 0.95 * 0.20 = 0.011145596, the first number on the dd line.

Table 7.17   Calculation of the probability of each possible parental phase in Figure 7.12 based upon the genotypes of the two affected children

| | Potential Paternal Phase | | | |
| | (only disease-bearing chromosome shown) | | | |
	A1-d-B1	A1-d-B2	A2-d-B1	A2-d-B2
Prior probability	0.25	0.25	0.25	0.25
II-1 A1-d	0.95	0.95	0.05	0.05
d-B2	0.20	0.80	0.20	0.80
II-2 A1-d	0.95	0.95	0.05	0.05
d-B2	0.20	0.80	0.20	0.80
Joint probability	0.009025000	0.144400000	0.000025000	0.000400000
Posterior probability	0.058661033	0.938576536	0.000162496	0.002599935

| | Potential Maternal Phase | | | |
| | (only disease-bearing chromosome shown) | | | |
	A3-d-B3	A3-d-B4	A4-d-B3	A4-d-B4
Prior probability	0.25	0.25	0.25	0.25
II-1 A4-d	0.05	0.05	0.95	0.95
d-B3	0.80	0.20	0.80	0.20
II-2 A4-d	0.05	0.05	0.95	0.95
d-B3	0.80	0.20	0.80	0.20
Joint probability	0.000400000	0.000025000	0.144400000	0.009025000
Posterior probability	0.002599935	0.000162496	0.938576536	0.058661033

Note: To conserve space or for simplicity of presentation, rounded numbers may be shown during the calculation. However, the unrounded, original numbers were used to calculate the final answer.

7.3   Single Markers and Potentially New Mutations

7.3.1   X-linked Inheritance

There are no true phase-known pedigrees when there is the possibility of a new mutation; the closest we can get is a pedigree that is phase-known for the DNA marker. Figure 7.13 shows the family of a phase-known (with respect to the marker locus) mother of an isolated affected male. Let us assume that $f = 0.5$, in which case the population frequency of female carriers will be 10μ (Table 2.10). The mother, II-1, is contemplating having more children and wants to know if we

Table 7.18   Calculation of the risk for II-3 in Figure 7.12 based upon the
probability of each possible parental phase

---

dd   = (0.011145596 + 0.713318167 + 0.000001625 + 0.000103997) *
       (0.000493988 + 0.000123497 + 0.009385765 + 0.002346441)
     = (0.724569385) * (0.012349691) = 0.008948208   affected

Nd   = (0.002346441 + 0.009385765 + 0.000123497 + 0.000493988) *
       (0.000493988 + 0.000123497 + 0.009385765 + 0.002346441)
     = (0.012349691) * (0.012349691) = 0.000152515   carrier

dN   = (0.011145596 + 0.713318167 + 0.000001625 + 0.000103997) *
       (0.000103997 + 0.000001625 + 0.713318167 + 0.011145596)
     = (0.724569385) * (0.724569385) = 0.525000794   carrier

NN   = (0.002346441 + 0.009385765 + 0.000123497 + 0.000493988) *
       (0.000103997 + 0.000001625 + 0.713318167 + 0.011145596)
     − (0.012349691) * (0.724569385) − 0.008948208   noncarrier

Total risk affected = 0.008948208 = 1.65%
Total risk carrier   = 0.525153309 = 96.70%
Total risk noncarrier = 0.008948208 = 1.65%

Note: To conserve space or for simplicity of presentation, rounded numbers may be
shown during the calculation. However, the unrounded, original numbers were used to
calculate the final answer.

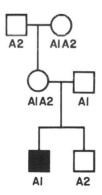

Figure 7.13   A family with an isolated case of an X-linked recessive disease (negative family history). Marker locus A is linked to the disease locus at $\theta = 0.02$. Assume that the disease in this family is not genetically lethal and that affected individuals have a reproductive fitness (f) of 0.5. The grandfather, I-1, is known to be
healthy. The probability of this pedigree is calculated in Table 7.19 and the carrier risks for I-2 and II-1 are discussed in the text.

Table 7.19 Calculation of the probabilities of combinations of genotypes in Figure 7.13

I-2 =	Carrier				Noncarrier		
Genotype =	A1-d/A2-N		A1-N/A2-d		A1-N/A2-N		
Prior risk	5μ		5μ		1		
II-1 =	C	NC	C	NC	C	C	NC
Genotype =	A1-d	A1-N	A1-d	A1-N	A1-d	A2-d	
	0.98	0.02	0.02	0.98	μ	ν	1
III-1 = A1-d	0.98	μ	0.98	μ	0.98	0.02	μ
III-2 = A2-N	0.98	1	0.98	1	0.98	0.02	1
Joint probability	4.706μ	$0.1\mu^2$	0.096μ	$4.9\mu^2$	0.96μ	0.0004ν	μ

Note: C = carrier, NC = noncarrier.

can determine her risks. Marker locus A recombines with the disease 2% of the time. The prior risk for I-2 is 10μ, which has to be divided equally between two potential phases, since no information is available on her father. If II-1 is a carrier, her phase can be only A1-d/A2-N if she inherited the mutation from her mother. If her mother is a noncarrier, the prior probability of A1-d is μ and the prior probability of A2-dis is ν.

I-2 is a carrier in columns 1 to 4 of Table 7.19. II-1 is a carrier in columns 1, 3, 5, and 6. If we ignore columns containing μ^2 and assume that $\mu = \nu$, the following risks are obtained:

I-2 = (4.706 + 0.096)/(4.706 + 0.096 + 0.96 + 0.0004 + 1)
   = (4.802)/(6.7624) = 0.71 = 71%
II-1 = (4.706 + 0.096 + 0.96 + 0.0004)/(6.7624)
   = (5.7624)/(6.7624) = 0.85 = 85%

To answer the original question about the prospects for the next child, we need to know how the potential risk is distributed between her two X chromosomes and what risk will be associated with the inheritance of either marker allele. Her carrier risk of 85% is almost exclusively associated with the maternal A1 chromosome, 5.762/5.7624 = 0.9999306, and 0.0004/5.7624 = 0.0000694 for the paternal A2 chromosome. The risk to a child inheriting an A1 allele will therefore be approximately 85 * 0.98 = 83.3%.

In Figure 7.14, the mother, I-1, is phase-unknown with respect to both the marker and the disease locus. This actually turns out to be a

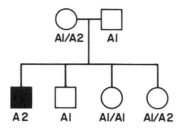

Figure 7.14   A two-generation family (phase unknown at both marker and disease loci) with an isolated case of an X-linked recessive disease. $\theta_A = 0.05$; $f = 0.7$. The risk that I-1 is a carrier is calculated in Table 7.20, and the risk that II-3 is a carrier is calculated in Table 7.21.

Table 7.20   Calculation of the carrier risk for I-1 in Figure 7.14

	Carrier		Noncarrier
Prior risk	18μ		1
Phase =	A1-dis/A2-NOR	A1-NOR/A2-dis	
Prior probability	0.5	0.5	1
II-1 (A2-dis)	0.05	0.95	μ
II-2 (A1-NOR)	0.05	0.95	1
Joint probability	0.0225μ	8.1225μ	μ
Total		8.14μ	μ
Risk		89.1%	10.9%

much easier calculation. The recombination fraction is 0.05 and the reproductive fitness is 0.7. When $f = 0.7$, the prior risk for I-1 is 18μ, which, since I-1 is phase-unknown, must be split equally between the two potential phases (Table 7.20).

Note that the carrier risk for I-1 (89.1%) is only marginally lower than the pedigree-only risk for the mother of an isolated affected male and no normal son (90%). This is because there is very little reduction for having a normal son with the opposite genotype than the affected male. In Bayesian calculations, the reduction of risk by normal sons is based upon the assumption that they have an equal opportunity to inherit the mutation if the mother is a carrier; when DNA testing tells us that this is not so because he probably inherited the opposite maternal X chromosome, the only reduction permitted is that which allows for the possibility that one or both of them is recombinant. The carrier risk for the first daughter, II-3, is calculated from the posterior proba-

Table 7.21   Calculation of the risk for II-3 in Figure 7.14

Phase in I-1 =	A1-dis/A2-NOR		A1-NOR/A2-dis		Noncarrier	
Conditional probability	0.0225		8.1225		1	
II-3 =	C	NC	C	NC	C	NC
(A1-?)	0.95	0.05	0.05	0.95	2μ	1
Joint probability	0.021375	0.001125	0.406125	7.716375	2μ	1
						(ignore)

Carrier total for II-3 = 0.021375 + 0.406125 = 0.4275
Noncarrier total for II-3 = 0.001125 + 7.716375 + 1.0 = 8.7175
   Total = 9.1450

Carrier = 0.4275/9.1450 = 4.675%
Noncarrier = 8.7175/9.1450 – 95.325%

Note: C = carrier, NC = noncarrier.

bility of each potential genotype in Table 7.21. For II-4, with opposite maternal genotype, the same numbers are added in a different way.

Carrier total   = 0.001125 + 7.716375   = 7.7175
Noncarrier total = 0.021375 + 0.406125 + 1.0 = 1.4275
 Total   9.1450
Carrier risk   = 7.7175/9.1450 – 0.8439, or 84.39%
Noncarrier risk = 1.4275/9.1450 = 0.1561, or 15.61%

The next example shows not only the contrast between how the calculation proceeds (in parallel) for almost identical (marker locus) phase-known and phase-unknown pedigrees but also that apparently very simple pedigrees can require some very complex thought.

In Figure 7.15, the disease is hemophilia A, which we will assume has a reproductive fitness of $f = 0.7$, which (assuming $\mu = \nu$) in turn gives a population carrier frequency of 18μ (see Table 2.10 or equation 2.4). The DNA polymorphism recombines with the disease locus 5% of the time (Table 7.22).

The result is certainly surprising at first appearance, since the risk is higher when the grandfather has not been tested (B) than when he has been tested (A) and he has the opposite allele to that found in his granddaughter. In the latter case (A), however, we now know that the granddaughter has inherited the grandmaternal X, whereas in the for-

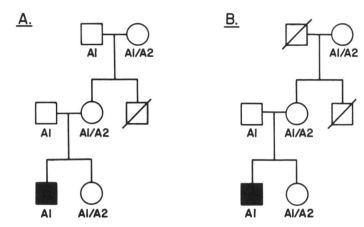

Figure 7.15 The paternal bottleneck. In both families the grandfather, I-1, was known not to have the hemophilia A found in his grandson (an isolated case). When the grandfather was available for testing with marker A ($\theta_A = 0.05$), the carrier risk for III-2 is higher than when he was not available for testing. Conversely, the carrier risk for II-2 is higher when her father was not available for testing than when he was (Table 7.22). This interesting phenomenon is caused by the apportioning of risk due to new mutations and inherited mutations between the two X chromosomes in II-2. When we have tested her father, we know which of her chromosomes is derived from him, and the mutational burden that this chromosome can carry is restricted (hence the bottleneck) because it was not mutant in him.

mer example there was the possibility that she might have inherited the grandpaternal X. The fact that there can be only a risk of 1μ (technically, 1ν) associated with the grandpaternal X chromosome after its transmission to the mother, when we know which one is his, I call the paternal bottleneck.

7.3.2 Autosomal Dominant Inheritance

There are relatively few useful applications for DNA markers in the case of an isolated affected individual with normal parents. Examples might be to offer some form of exclusion testing if a suitable family structure is available (e.g., if both parents are heterozygous at the marker locus and the affected child homozygous) or partial confirmation of the likelihood of the affected having homozygous normal parents if penetrance < 1.0 and there are sufficient healthy siblings with the same marker alleles as the affected. Direct mutation testing is the only viable option in many situations.

7.3.3 Autosomal Recessive Inheritance

Autosomal recessive inheritance is also a nonapplication, since if there was some way to prove that one parent was a definite noncarrier of the recessive disorder, why do any further testing (besides trying to prove a non-Mendelian mode of transmission in this family)? If the child is homozygous for all loci tested, the pedigree should be studied carefully with uniparental disomy in mind. Almost all autosomal recessive pedigrees with only one affected child would look the same if that child had a new mutation or had two carrier parents.

7.4   Flanking Markers and Potentially New Mutations

7.4.1 X-linked Inheritance

As in the section on single-side markers, there are no truly phase-known pedigrees in potential new mutation situations. Figure 7.16 shows the analysis of a small family with a lethal X-linked recessive disease ($f = 0$).

If θ_A and θ_B are both equal to 0.10, we would expect the following categories of meioses

No crossovers $= 0.9 * 0.9$ $= 0.81$
Single crossovers $= 2 * 0.9 * 0.1 = 0.18$ (0.09 each)
Double crossovers $= 0.1 * 0.1$ $= 0.01$

When the mother is a carrier, she has four potential phases, the probability of which we determine based upon the evidence at hand (her affected son) (Table 7.23). However, the mother will be a carrier only 2/3 of the time, so the final risks are calculated as shown in Table 7.24.

7.4.2 Autosomal Dominant Inheritance

The same comments apply here as in section 7.3.2.

7.4.3 Autosomal Recessive Inheritance

See section 7.3.3 for comments.

7.5   Direct Detection of Mutations

Although there are obvious exceptions, for the last several years, a general time-course for the cloning of genes and elucidation of muta-

Table 7.22 Calculation of the carrier risk for III-2 in Figure 7.15 (A and B): influence of the availability of the maternal grandfather

	Grandfather Tested			Grandfather Not Tested		
I-2 =	Carrier (18μ)		Noncarrier	Carrier (18μ)		Noncarrier
	A1h/A2H	A1H/A2h	A1H/A2H	A1h/A2H	A1H/A2h	A1H/A2H
Prior probability	9μ	9μ	1	9μ	9μ	1
Son II-3	0.5	0.5	1	0.5	0.5	1
Posterior probability	4.5μ	4.5μ	1	4.5μ	4.5μ	1
II-2 =	A1h/A2H	A1H/A2h	A1H/A2H	A1h/A2H	A1H/A2h	A1H/A2H
Old mutation	0†	4.5μ‡	1	2.25μ	2.25μ	1
New mutation	1μ	1μ	0	1μ	1μ	0
Total	1μ	5.5μ	1μ	3.25μ§	3.25μ	1μ
III-1 = A1-h	0.95	0.05	1μ	0.95	0.05	1μ
Joint probability	0.95	0.275	1	3.0875	0.1625	1
Posterior probability	42.7%	12.4%	44.9%	72.65%	3.82%	23.53%

III-2 =	C	NC	C	NC	C	NC
Phase in II-2	42.7	44.9	12.4	72.65	3.82	23.53
DNA A1H/A2?	0.05	1	0.95	0.05	0.95	1
Joint probability	2.135	44.9 +40.57‖ +0.62#	11.7	3.63	3.63	23.53 +69.01¶ +0.19††
Posterior probability	2.135%	86.09%	11 78%	3.63%	3.63%	92.74%
Total	13.9%	86.1%		7.3%		92.7%

†0.00 with the maternal A2 marker, since she is not affected (A1h/A2h). In this column, we are calculating the risk that the A1 that she inherited from her father is associated with a new mutation.

‡4.5μ with the maternal marker A2 (actually [4.5μ * 0.95] from a maternal A2h plus [4.5μ * 0.05] from a maternal A1h). The 1μ under new mutations would also be with the maternal A2.

§This could be 2.25μ with a maternal A1 and an additional 1μ either with a maternal A1 (total 3.25μ for A1) or a paternal A2 (total A1 2.25μ/A2 1μ). We cannot distinguish between the various possibilities, but the total for both carrier columns will eventually become 3.25μ for both A1 and A2 by a process similar to that shown in note B.

‖42.7 * 0.95 = +40.57

¶72.65 * 0.95 = +69.01

#12.4 * 0.05 = +0.62

††3.82 * 0.05 = +0.19

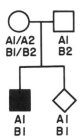

Figure 7.16   A family with a negative family history of a genetically lethal X-linked recessive disease. Marker loci A and B flank the disease locus at θ_A = 0.10 and θ_B = 0.10. The probabilities of the four potential maternal phases are calculated in Table 7.23 and then combined with the probability that the mother is a carrier to determine the risk to the fetus (Table 7.24).

Table 7.23   Risk to II-2 in Figure 7.16 when the mother is a carrier

Maternal Phase	Affected Son = A1-d-B1	Risk That Fetus = A1-d-B1	Risk That Fetus = A1-N-B1
A1-d-B1	0.81 *	0.81 = 0.6561	0.01 = 0.0081
A1-d-B2	0.09 *	0.09 = 0.0081	0.09 = 0.0081
A2-d-B1	0.09 *	0.09 = 0.0081	0.09 = 0.0081
A2-d-B2	0.01 *	0.01 = 0.0001	0.81 = 0.0081
Total		0.6724	0.0324
		95.4% (affected)	4.6% (normal)

Note: To conserve space or for simplicity of presentation, rounded numbers may be shown during the calculation. However, the unrounded, original numbers were used to calculate the final answer.

tions causing diseases might be (1) linkage is detected between the disease and a DNA marker, (2) flanking markers are identified, giving a candidate region, (3) positional cloning methods identify a candidate cDNA, and (4) mutations are found in the gene or its control regions which can explain the disease phenotype.

This book deals mostly with the theory of the diagnostic aspects available during the first two stages of this process (and in the case of intragenic polymorphisms, the third stage). Once the fourth stage has been reached, very little general theory is needed because the answers provided by the laboratory tests will normally be absolute (assuming Mendelian inheritance). However, this presumes that it is economically feasible to provide the tests that have 100% accuracy to large numbers of people. The fourth stage, although technologically feasible

Table 7.24 Risk for II-2 in Figure 7.16 allowing for the possibility that II-1 has a new mutation

Mother =	Carrier		Noncarrier	
Posterior risk	0.667		0.333	
Fetus =	Affected	Normal	Affected	Normal
Conditional probability	0.954	0.046	μ	1
Joint probability	0.636	0.031	Ignore	0.333

Posterior risk affected = 63.6%
Posterior risk normal = 36.4%

in many instances, in the early 1990s is actually applied in relatively few. As an example, the factor VIII gene involved in hemophilia A was among the first of the major human disease genes to be cloned and sequenced (1983); ten years later, a few research laboratories attempt to detect the specific mutations in this gene in hemophilia A, but true diagnostic laboratories cannot afford to attempt this on a routine basis. In 1990–91, the factor IX gene from many of our hemophilia B patients was sequenced in S. Sommer's laboratory (Koeberl et al. 1991). In some cases, a restriction enzyme was identified that could detect the mutation directly, but in most familial cases, even when we knew the mutation, the cost of mutation analysis in additional family members would far exceed the cost of providing the answer by PCR analysis of intragenic polymorphisms.

The direct detection of mutations becomes much more feasible when one or a small number of specific mutations cause the disease, as in the common mutation for cystic fibrosis or in the mutation causing sickle cell anemia. In such cases, following a positive result, calculations are not necessary since the test result is specific. It is worth pointing out, however, that my personal experience in direct mutation testing for cystic fibrosis has been disappointing so far. Despite testing for more mutations than most other laboratories (e.g., 20 mutations in mid-1992), I have found fewer cases than expected where both mutations could be identified. Commercial laboratories tend to perform a standard panel of tests that can be applied cheaply and reproducibly; if these tests are uninformative, no further tests are offered. This approach is fundamentally different from that used in an academic setting, where some attempt is made to provide useful information to help every family. An academic center would likely start with the same tests as the commercial laboratory but, in the event that these do not help, should have a substantial repertoire of other tests that can be tried until an answer is found. Clearly, linkage and linkage disequilibrium studies will be valuable adjuncts for a long time, even for diseases in which direct mutation testing holds so much promise.

Whenever a high proportion of cases is due to new mutation, the search for frequent mutations will prove fruitless unless an unusual feature is present in the DNA that generates a mutational "hot spot." Thus there is little point in searching for frequent mutations in genetically lethal X-linked recessive diseases, because almost every family will have a different mutation (the proportion of this book devoted to X-linked conditions under conditions where a new mutation might be present is no accident). An example of an exception to this rule is fragile X syndrome, where the majority of mutations are confined to an extremely small region, and there is an easy method to screen for them (it is effectively a genetic lethal in affected males, but not in male carriers of a "premutation"). Fragile X syndrome may also be an exception to the rule that we do not normally detect linkage disequilibrium in association with X-linked diseases. Similarly, in Duchenne muscular dystrophy, because a large proportion (2/3) of cases have easily detectable deletions, the search for these is useful (the remaining 1/3 still expect an answer, however, which must involve the use of polymorphisms or other tests).

It is relevant to note at this point that the pattern of mutations in any given gene often seems to change with time. Initial reports of mutations frequently refer to mutations that are unusually easy to detect. Only after many mutations have been characterized by sequence analysis do we eventually determine the true pattern (and since it is often difficult to publish papers reporting the thirtieth or the ninetieth point mutation at a no-longer-novel genetic locus, we frequently have to wait for reviews that summarize known mutations). As examples, early papers reporting the characterization of mutations causing hemophilia A, hemophilia B, and Hunter syndrome (all X-linked recessive disorders) almost universally reported large deletions. It would be an error, however, to assume that the major mechanism of mutation at these loci is by large genomic deletion, as in a large proportion of cases of Duchenne muscular dystrophy. Instead, we are seeing a bias in the first few papers that reflects the ease of detection of large deletions. Duchenne muscular dystrophy is an exception: most other loci probably have deletions or insertions as the mechanism of mutation in only 5% to 10% of cases. A similar bias, although to a lesser extent, is often also seen in the initial reporting of mutations that create or destroy a site for specific restriction enzymes (e.g., Taq I and Msp I) within the coding sequence. Like the deletions, these mutations are relatively easy to detect and so tend to be reported first; they are not necessarily the most common.

As the "Genome Project" continues, a great deal of valuable information will become available, which will change how we perform analyses for specific diseases. There is nothing new in this, however; until we reach the stage of true "reverse genetics" rather than the current "positional cloning," it will merely increase the pace at which diseases will transit from first linked marker to direct detection of mutations, and for every disease nearing the end of this process several more will probably be just beginning. Only when a disease can be tested exclusively by mutation analysis will the need for risk calculations disappear altogether (e.g., sickle cell disease). For the next ten years, there will be a great increase in information pertaining to DNA markers, linkage maps, cDNA sequences, etc. The complete primary sequence is scheduled to be available in the early part of next century. If we are to reap the maximum medical benefits from this work, it will be necessary to apply what we know to the general population now, and with notable exceptions, cost currently precludes us from offering personal DNA sequence analysis or direct mutation testing.

7.6   Uniparental Disomy

Uniparental disomy is defined as the inheritance of two homologous chromosomes from the same parent. In the absence of a trisomy, it also implies a lack of inheritance of a homologue from the other parent. Although the basic term refers to complete normal chromosomes, variants of the basic mechanism might extend to partial regional disomies comprising structurally abnormal chromosomes or partial regional disomies resulting from an exchange of part of the genetic material between structurally normal chromosomes such that all copies of particular genes or chromosomal regions are derived from the same bivalent chromosome in only one parent. If the two homologues are identical, uniparental homodisomy or isodisomy has occurred; if the two homologues are different, uniparental heterodisomy has occurred.

This cytogenetic description is, unfortunately, a gross oversimplification. Recombination makes the molecular genetic interpretation of disomy much more difficult. Clinicians should be interested in the molecular ramifications of recombination, since exactly the same arguments apply to the inheritance of single disease-causing loci as to the inheritance of single marker loci.

Let us briefly review meiotic nondisjunction involving the X and Y chromosomes in male meiosis. Just before the first meiotic division, each of these chromosomes will be present in the cell as a bivalent that contains two identical DNA molecules joined at the centromere, that is, two copies of each gene on the X chromosome packaged into a single structure called a bivalent and two copies of each gene on the Y chromosome packaged into the other bivalent. During the first meiotic division, the bivalent X chromosome should go into one product and the Y chromosome bivalent into the other. Each bivalent still has two DNA molecules containing two full sets of all the genes on either the X or the Y chromosome, so we have a "2X cell" and a "2Y cell." During the second meiotic division, the centromere of each bivalent should be broken, and a single DNA molecule containing a haploid set of all the X chromosome genes or all the Y chromosome genes is placed into each of the four product cells that will eventually become sperm (Figure 7.17). Nondisjunction can occur at either of these two steps. Meiotic nondisjunction 1 (NDJ-1) (Figure 7.18) leads to both the X and the Y chromosomes bivalent being placed in the same "cell" (failure to pull the centromeres to opposite poles). Now one "cell" has all four DNA molecules (two sets of X and two sets of Y chromosome genes), while the other has none (ignoring the autosomes in this simplified description).

During the second division, the centromere of each bivalent breaks, and one of the DNA molecules should be pulled to each pole, resulting eventually in two "cells," each containing a complete set of X chromosome genes and a complete set of Y chromosome genes. If these sperm fuse with a normal ovum, a 47,XXY karyotype would result, causing Klinefelter syndrome. NDJ-I leads to dissimilar chromosomes being found in the sperm (cytogenetic heterodisomy). NDJ-II (Figure 7.18) would result from a failure to pull apart the two haploid sets of genes at the time that the centromere of the bivalent should break, so both sets of X chromosome genes or both sets of Y chromosome genes end up in the same sperm. In this case the sperm would contain similar sex chromosomes (cytogenetic homodisomy) and would lead to either 47,XXX or 47,XYY offspring, depending upon whether it was disomic for the X or the Y.

NDJ-I leads to two nullisomic gametes and two heterodisomic gametes; NDJ-II leads to two normal gametes, one nullisomic and one homodisomic gamete (Table 7.25). So far, so good; now let us make things more complex by considering chromosomal homologues where recombination can occur and where we need to trace the progress of particular loci through the meiotic divisions. It turns out that nondisjunction at either meiotic division can yield either homozygosity or heterozygosity for a specific locus, depending upon whether or not the

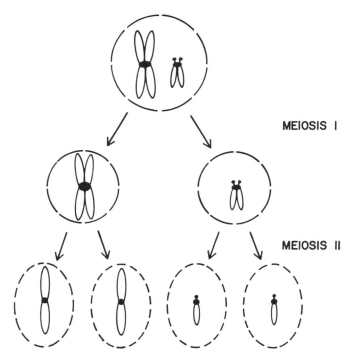

MEIOSIS I

MEIOSIS II

Figure 7.17   The normal segregation of the X and Y chromosomes during male meiosis. The bivalents shown at the top have two complete DNA molecules held together at the centromere. In the first meiotic division the two members of the pair of homologues are separated. During the second meiotic division the centromeres of the bivalents break (in the vertical plane in this diagram) and a single complete DNA molecule is packaged into each gamete. The *dashed line* around the chromosomes is for illustrative purposes; no defined nucleus is present during the meiotic divisions.

breakpoint occurred between the centromere and that locus and, in the case of NDJ-I, the specific assortment of the chromatids during the second division. In Figures 7.19 and 7.20, showing NDJ-I and NDJ-II following recombination, it can be seen that NDJ-I can lead to homozygosity for loci distal to the breakpoint (same color) in the first pattern of segregation of the chromatids, and to heterozygosity for any locus or region of the chromosome (one black plus one white). The second pattern of segregation leads only to heterozygosity in Figure 7.19, although multiple crossover events involving all chromatids might change that. NDJ-II will lead to distal heterozygosity instead. Although Figures 7.19 and 7.20 show only a single breakpoint, in a series of meioses, there will actually be a gradient of increased homozygosity or heterozygosity diverging away from the centromere, de-

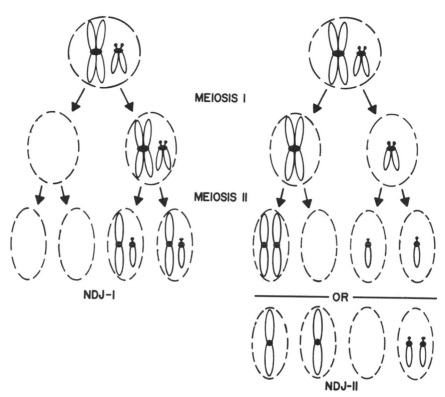

Figure 7.18   Nondisjunction of the X and Y chromosomes during male meiosis. Nondisjunction in the first meiotic division (*NDJ-I*) is shown on the *left* and non-disjunction in the second meiotic division (*NDJ-II*) is shown on the *right*. NDJ-I leads to two gametes containing two dissimilar chromosomes (heterodisomic) and to two nullisomic gametes. NDJ-II leads to one gamete containing two similar chromosomes (homodisomic), one nullisomic and two normal gametes.

Table 7.25   Segregation of chromatids during normal division and during nondisjunction in male meiosis

	Prophase	Anaphase I	Anaphase II
Normal	XX YY	XX YY	X X Y Y
NDJ-I	XX YY	XX YY O	XY XY O O
NDJ-II	XX YY	XX YY	XX O Y Y or
			X X YY O

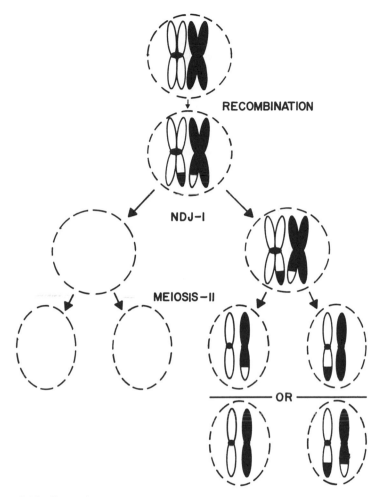

Figure 7.19   Recombination followed by nondisjunction in the first meiotic division (*NDJ-I*) can lead to homozygosity (*same color*) for regions distal to the breakpoint or to no apparent deviation from heterozygosity (*bottom*), depending upon the segregation of the chromatids during the second meiotic division.

pending upon which division the nondisjunction event occurred in. This approach has been used to study the origin of chromosomes and the division in which nondisjunction occurred in trisomy 21 by Sherman et al. (1991).

If the contributory parent is homozygous for the polymorphisms studied, the disomy will escape detection in the molecular laboratory unless the other noncontributory parent has different alleles, and a lack of their inheritance is noted. If the contributory parent is heterozygous,

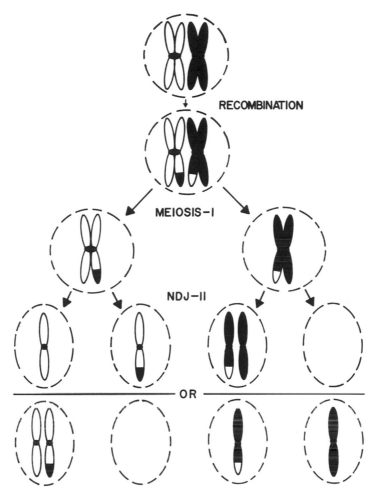

Figure 7.20 Recombination followed by nondisjunction in the second meiotic divison (*NDJ-II*) leads to homozygosity at loci proximal to the breakpoint and to heterozygosity at loci distal to the breakpoint in the disomic gamete.

homodisomy and heterodisomy will yield different genotypes in the child (homozygous and heterozygous); again, detection depends upon the noncontributory parent's having a genotype that is noted to be absent. One conclusion that all of this leads to is that apparent nonpaternity should not be dismissed as true nonpaternity without further thought. Apparent nonmaternity, of course, is never summarily dismissed.

If disomy is detected, the consequence to the child depends upon whether it is homodisomy or heterodisomy, the mode of inheritance of the disorder, the carrier status of the contributory parent, and whether or not chromosomal imprinting is relevant to gene expression for the region involved. As an extreme example of why apparent non-paternity should be carefully evaluated, it is possible that a carrier mother for an X-linked disease could have an affected female fetus through maternal homodisomy; to presume that the "biological father" contributed the opposite allele to that identified in the husband would be disastrous. A recombination event associated with uniparental disomy might also alter the phase of loci susceptible to *cis-trans* positional effects (section 1.7) even without apparently affecting overall heterozygosity.

It might well be that uniparental heterodisomy occurs quite frequently and without much consequence; similarly, uniparental homodisomy might be relatively frequent but escape detection because the contributory parent was not a carrier of a recessive disease located on the chromosome or in the chromosomal region passed in double dose. It is obviously important to molecular genetics laboratories to find out the actual frequency of non-Mendelian inheritance, since so much rides on the presumed parental origin of each allele.

7.7   Genetic Heterogeneity

In Figure 7.21, prenatal diagnosis has been requested for an autosomal dominant condition where there is known to be genetic heterogeneity. There are at least two clinically indistinguishable forms of this disease; one form, which accounts for 90% of cases, is linked to a marker that recombines 2% of the time; the remaining cases are unlinked to this marker. This disease shows 70% penetrance.

II-1 is phase-known A1-nor/A2-DIS *if* the disease is caused by the common locus that is linked to the marker. In the remaining 10% of cases, the marker information is irrelevant, and the prior risk is 50% (Table 7.26). For the common locus, the fetus has inherited the paternal A1 allele, which was coupled to the normal allele. It will have the mutation only if it is recombinant. Note that following the DNA analysis, the risk is about three times greater that the fetus will be affected by the rarer form of the disease.

7.8   Linkage Disequilibrium and Haplotype Analysis

When two loci are closely linked, a phenomenon known as linkage disequilibrium might be noted when certain conditions are met. For

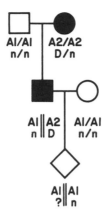

Figure 7.21   A family with a positive family history of a fully penetrant but hetero-geneous autosomal dominant disease. Marker locus A is linked at θ = 0.02 to the form of the disease that accounts for 90% of cases. The remaining 10% of cases are clinically indistinguishable but exhibit no linkage to this marker. The family is phase-known only if the disease locus in this family is the one that is linked to marker locus A.

Table 7.26   Calculation of risk for an autosomal dominant condition in which genetic heterogeneity is known to occur (Fig. 7.21)

	Linked?			
	Yes = 0.9		No = 0.1	
	A1-DIS	A1-nor	DIS	nor
Conditional probability	0.02	0.98	0.5	0.5
Joint probability	0.018.	0.882	0.05	0.05

Total DIS = 0.068
Total nor = 0.932

Probability of being affected = 0.068 * 0.7 = 0.0476 (4.76%)
Probability of being unaffected = 0.9524 (95.24%)
(Probability of being nonpenetrant carrier = 0.0204, or 2.04%)

two closely linked loci with alleles A1/A2 and B1/B2, the frequency at equilibrium with which the four haplotypes, A1-B1, A1-B2, A2-B1, and A2-B2, would be expected to occur in the general population is the product of the individual allele frequencies. Thus, if A1 and A2 have frequencies of 0.7 and 0.3, and B1 and B2 have frequencies of 0.9 and 0.1, we would expect

A1-B1 = 0.7 * 0.9 = 0.63
A1-B2 = 0.7 * 0.1 = 0.07
A2-B1 = 0.3 * 0.9 = 0.27
A2-B2 = 0.3 * 0.1 = 0.03
Total   1.00

These are population statistics. In any given family, the loci will obviously be linked at θ_{AB}, and the presence of a particular allele at the A locus will be strongly predictive of which B allele is present.

If we could travel back to a time before the B locus became polymorphic (e.g., all chromosomes are B1 because the mutation that causes the B2 allele has not yet occurred), we would have only two haplotypes, A1-B1 (0.7) and A2-B1 (0.3). When a B1 allele mutates to become the first B2, it must do so on either an A1 or an A2 chromosome, say, A1. Initially, B2 will be found exclusively in the A1-B2 haplotype, and the distribution of haplotypes might be

A1-B1 = 0.69
A1-B2 = 0.01
A2-B1 = 0.30
A2-B2 = 0.00

Since we currently are aware of the B locus because it is polymorphic, the frequency of the B2 allele obviously increased in the population. This in itself, however, will not lead to four haplotypes at equilibrium frequencies. To generate the A2-B2 haplotype requires recombination between the two loci in the relatively rare doubly heterozygous individuals. After many generations and recombination events, equilibrium will be established. Disequilibrium will persist if θ is so small that the many recombination events required to establish equilibrium have not yet occurred or if the new allele was generated so recently that equilibrium has not yet been reached (sometimes even when θ is relatively large). Linkage disequilibrium is therefore a manifestation of genetic propinquity—nearness in either place or time.

If the mutation at the B locus causes disease instead of being a harmless polymorphism, we may be able to use linkage disequilibrium in a predictive sense in instances where conventional linkage testing does not apply or cannot be performed. As an example, I shall describe how linkage disequilibrium has been applied to some families concerned about cystic fibrosis. Beaudet et al. (1989) studied the association between cystic fibrosis and normal chromosomes and certain haplotypes at the D7S23 locus (alleles at the XV-2c and KM-19 sites). They determined the frequency with which four haplotypes, A to D, were found to be associated with normal and cystic fibrosis chromo-

somes. From these data it is possible to derive two useful statistics;
(a) the probability that a chromosome bearing a given haplotype also
has a mutation causing cystic fibrosis and (b) the probability that individuals with a given genotype (pair of haplotypes) will be carriers of
cystic fibrosis. They found that the B haplotype occurred on cystic
fibrosis chromosomes with a frequency of 0.0173 and on normal chromosomes with a frequency of 0.137. The probability that a random
chromosome with the B haplotype carries the disease is therefore
0.0173/(0.0173 + 0.137) = 0.0173/0.1543 = 0.112 (11.2% or odds of
1 in 8.9). The results for the A, C, and D haplotypes were 0.0046,
0.0013, and 0.0062, respectively, which clearly illustrates the very
strong association of cystic fibrosis with the B haplotype. The probability that an individual with a BD genotype is a carrier is given by the
sum of the two individual probabilities minus twice the product of
these probabilities (because the individual is known not to be affected)
= 0.112 + 0.0062 − (2 ∗ 0.112 ∗ 0.0062) = 0.1182 − (0.0013888) =
0.1168 (11.7% or odds of 1 in 8.5). The highest carrier risk is obviously
for a person with a BB genotype (20% risk). Genotypes containing one
B have carrier risks of approximately 11 to 12%, most genotypes without a B have a carrier risk of 1% or less. (Ethnic note: these figures
apply to those of European origin only; Asian families and North
American black families were not included in this analysis. Estivill
et al. (1988) reported a similar study in Italian families.)

Before mutation testing was available for cystic fibrosis, haplotype-
based risks were the only way to modify the carrier risk of someone
marrying into a cystic fibrosis family. As an example, suppose that the
healthy sibling of someone who died of cystic fibrosis wanted to know
the chance that she and her new spouse might have an affected child.
If the affected person died before any linkage or other test could be
performed, we could use population statistics (carrier frequency = 1/
25) to guide them (2/3 ∗ 1/25 ∗ 1/4 = 1/150), but it is likely that testing
their haplotypes will provide more specific information. For instance,
if she had a genotype containing one or two B haplotypes, her carrier
risk would increase; if her spouse had a BB genotype, his risk would
increase from 1/25 to 1/5, whereas, if he had a CC genotype, it would
drop to 1/384.

In small families where it was not possible to test the affected individual but all other members were available to test, it might still have
been possible to perform an indirect linkage test based upon the probable genotype of the affected child. For instance, parents with genotypes AB and BD probably donated the two B haplotypes to their
affected child. A calculation similar to that in Table 7.5 could be envi-
sioned where the probability of phase was obtained from the relative

likelihoods of the disease being associated with the B haplotype or the non-B haplotypes and then using the recombination fraction between D7S23 and cystic fibrosis to complete the table.

Although the cystic fibrosis gene has now been cloned, and more than 200 mutations have been characterized (perhaps surprising, since the detection of disequilibrium is to some extent dependent upon all cases being derived from one or very few common ancestors), the detection rate of mutations in affected individuals is still not 100%. As I can attest from personal experience, there are many requests made of a molecular laboratory "to rule out" cystic fibrosis in newborns. If the most frequent mutations are not present, linkage disequilibrium may reduce the remaining risk considerably more than testing a whole battery of additional mutations (with frequencies <1/200 each), and yet many would now consider such tests archaic.

As a cautionary note, linkage disequilibrium has been noted during the search for *some* disease loci. This neither guarantees that it will be noted during the search for all other disease-causing loci nor that, if found, the disease-causing locus must necessarily be extremely close. A particular problem may arise when investigators treat linkage disequilibrium and linkage as interchangeable processes and try to order genetic maps based upon linkage disequilibrium observations. I believe that the observation of, or the failure to observe, linkage disequilibrium may have led some investigators either to miss what is there or to imagine what isn't there. The necessary conditions for the observation of linkage disequilibrium are (a) the existence of polymorphism at both loci so that different forms can be discriminated and (b) the physical or the temporal proximity of the detectable polymorphisms.

Let me give two hypothetical examples. In the first example, a disease-causing locus exhibits linkage disequilibrium with two groups of polymorphisms that are known to be well separated on a genetic map. This is not a problem unless we start to think that the linkage map must be wrong because it apparently disagrees with the linkage disequilibrium data. In order to detect statistically significant linkage disequilibrium, it is likely that enough samples will have been studied to have given very high lod/location scores for the genetic map. There are, of course, potential explanations for the apparent discrepancy that do not involve the assumption that a linkage map with very high lod/location scores is incorrect. Why could there not be twin loci? Could there be a distant enhancer region? Could the two regions of disequilibrium bound the 5' and 3' ends of the gene? (polymorphism is mandatory for the detection of linkage disequilibrium, and polymorphism tends to occur less in the structural parts of genes (the middle) and more in the flanking, noncoding regions). Could the two pockets of linkage disequilibrium mean that almost all disease-causing mutations occur in two hot spots, one at either end of a large gene?

In the second example, let us assume that there are three loci, A, B, and C, in that order on the chromosome. Let us assume that loci A and B can have polymorphic alleles A1 or A2 and B1 or B2 and that locus C causes a dominant disease with alleles D (disease) or n (normal). If we travel back to a time when only locus A was polymorphic, all chromosomes had either the A1-B1-n or the A2-B1-n haplotype. If a disease-causing mutation occurred on a chromosome with allele A1 and then a second mutation occurred at the B locus soon afterward, A1-B1-D and A1-B2-D haplotypes now exist (the first being created by a mutation at the disease locus, and the second being created from the first by a subsequent mutation at the B locus). The haplotypes A2-B1-D and A2-B2-D will eventually arise by recombination between the A and B loci. The point is that it might be possible for locus B to be in apparent linkage equilibrium with the disease locus and locus A to be in apparent linkage disequilibrium even though it is actually more distant. This apparent discrepancy will fade with time as recombination takes place between the A locus and the other two, but caught at the right moment in evolution, it might provide a diversion for gene-hunters determined to find and act upon any hint of linkage disequilibrium.

7.9   When Do Mutations Occur?

Mutations presumably can occur in any cell at any time. Does it matter in which cell type and at what stage of the life cycle a particular mutation might occur? The answer is, of course, yes. All humans start as a single cell, the zygote. The human body contains something of the order of 10^{14} cells, which are all descended from this zygote. Given that many of the cells first descended from the zygote form the placenta and other structures rather than the actual embryo, it is reasonable to assume that an absolute minimum of 50 rounds of mitosis would be required to generate a "person" ($2^{46.5} = 10^{14}$). Not all of these cells are involved in gametogenesis, of course, and it has been estimated that approximately 23 rounds of mitosis would be required to produce the approximately 8 million oocytes present in female ovaries (however, only about 400 ova are ever released), and approximately 30 rounds to produce the sperm-producing cells of the seminiferous tubules (Wijsman 1991). There is a further major difference between gametogenesis in the different sexes: in females, once the oocytes have been formed, there is no need for ongoing mitotic activity; in contrast, in males, it has been estimated that spermatogenesis requires an additional 23 rounds of mitosis per year following its initiation at puberty. Sperm from an older male may therefore be the ultimate products of a much greater number of mitotic cell divisions before the final meiotic division than sperm from a younger male.

If the human mutation rate is $3.2 * 10^{-9}$ per base pair per generation (Koeberl et al. 1990), and there are 50,000 genes with a mean coding sequence of 1,200 bp, we would expect that one mutation of functional significance would be produced every five generations. Perhaps *fixed* would be a better word than *produced* in the previous sentence, because a mutant gamete needs to be fertilized and successfully expressed in the offspring before we notice it. The probability that any given gamete will become a baby is extremely low (approximately 1 in 20,000 potential ova are released, of which maybe 1 in 100 become children), and a miniscule fraction of sperm (made at a rate of approximately 1,000 per second, or 10^8 per day) ever become children. Given the mutation rate and the very large number of cells involved, we may conclude that all adult humans have within their gonads a large number of mutant gametes or potential gametes (including mutations for almost all genetic diseases) but that it is relatively rare to have one of these actually fertilized and the mutation recognized in the resultant offspring.

The question of relevance to the calculation of recurrence risks is not, what is the mutation rate, but, given that a new mutation has been found within the family, what is the probability that it will recur among further offspring of that parent. The answer depends upon when it occurred in the chain of events linking zygote to adult to gamete. Almost all of the calculations in other sections of this book assume that the mutation was present at the time of conception, so all cells in the body contain it and Mendelian risks apply. If the mutation occurred in the last step, meiosis, the recurrence risk (of the same mutation from that parent) is virtually 0 (but the risk to the offspring of the person who just inherited it will be the normal Mendelian risk); if it occurred early in the embryonic formation of the parent, so that all the gonadal tissue is mutant, the recurrence risk will equal the Mendelian risk, just as if the parent were a conventional carrier or were affected. If it occurred even earlier in embryogenesis, the parent may be a somatic mosaic as well as a gonadal mosaic and may show symptoms of the disease. But what if it happened at a stage such that only part of a gonad contains the mutation? The recurrence risk will be somewhere between 0 and the full Mendelian risk. The case of the gonadal mosaic ("partial carrier") is the most difficult to determine recurrence risks for.

Empirical studies on recurrence of new mutations for Duchenne muscular dystrophy have shown that the risk of recurrence is approximately 7% (or 14% if the person was phase-known and the "at-risk" haplotype is passed on again) (Bakker et al. 1989). Passos-Bueno et al. (1992) refined this analysis to include the nature of the mutation and concluded that deletions in the proximal hot spot of the dystrophin gene have a recurrence risk of 30% for the at-risk haplotype and deletions in the distal hot spot have a 4% recurrence risk for the at-risk haplotype (the recurrence risk of the at-risk haplotype for a conventional obligate carrier is 100%). The high recurrence risk of proximal deletions suggests that many of the mothers who have passed on such "new" mutations are gonadal mosaics and also that a high proportion of the gonad contains the mutation (i.e., the mutation probably resulted from a mitosis early in embryogenesis). The lower risk associated with the distal deletions perhaps indicates that these mutations are more likely to occur later in the embryonic development of the mother.

Duchenne muscular dystrophy is the best-characterized disease in relation to recurrence risks for apparently new mutations. For other diseases, it would seem very prudent to assume that the recurrence risk will also be of a similar magnitude under apparently new mutation situations (including cases where there is an apparently new mutation in a family with an autosomal recessive disease, e.g., White et al. 1991). If prenatal testing can be performed on subsequent offspring, its merits should be considered very seriously.

Whether mutations occur before or during gametogenesis (i.e., mitotic or meiotic) was also discussed in the last paragraph of section 6.2 in the context of models for incorporating new mutations into risk calculations. It is worth noting that some alleles contain more than one mutation. Koeberl et al. (1990) reported that the factor IX gene had two sequence alterations in 2 out of 26 families with hemophilia B. Whether these represent mutations occurring on different occasions or two mutations in response to a single environmental insult is not known.

8

Integration of RFLP Data
with Non-DNA Parameters

8.1 Biochemical Test Results

When we considered the introduction of biochemical test results into
Bayesian calculations, great emphasis was placed upon the difference
between linear and nonlinear predictors of risk. Recombination data
are linear, in that recombination is twice as likely to occur when $\theta =$
0.10 as when $\theta = 0.05$. To combine other types of data with RFLP
results, we should convert the other types of data to linear scales. By
this we mean specifically that the maximal value will be 1.0, the mini-
mal value will be 0.0, the midpoint will be 0.5, and someone with a
value of 0.8 is twice as likely to be a carrier as someone with a value
of 0.4.

8.1.1 Intragenic Polymorphisms

In Figure 8.1, we are considering the segregation of an X-linked
recessive condition and an intragenic polymorphism that is assumed
not to recombine with the disease-causing mutation. The mother is
heterozygous for both, but is phase-unknown. Her phase is either A1-
disease/A2-normal or A1-normal/A2-disease, but since both affected
males are deceased, we cannot use them to determine the correct
phase. Assume that she has three children, the affected male, a second
child represented by the diamond, and a daughter who wants to know
her carrier status. The daughter has a biochemical test result of 0.5,
which is not helpful. We are left with trying to determine the phase in
the mother by using the second child. Below the main pedigree, the

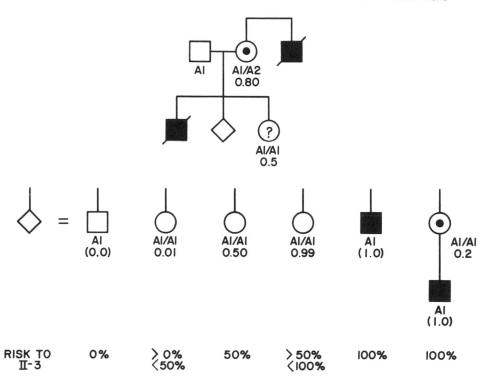

Figure 8.1 At the *top* of this figure is the pedigree of a phase-unknown family
with a positive family history of an X-linked recessive disease. Marker A is an intragenic polymorphism that we will assume never recombines with the disease
The numbers refer to the results of a biochemical test that can be used to predict carrier status (the numbers in brackets are the hypothetical values for affected and normal males). In the *lower half* of the figure, the influence of the
second child (represented by the *diamond*) upon the phase in the mother is considered for several different scenarios. At the *left*, the second child is assumed to
be an unaffected male with marker allele A1. He would allow us to determine
that the phase in his mother is definitely A1-N/A2-d, and so the risk that II-3 is a
carrier would become 0%. At the *right*, an affected male or an obligate carrier female with marker allele A1 would have exactly the opposite effect. In the *center*,
females with marker allele A1, but in whom we are not so certain of the genotype
at their disease locus, would have an effect intermediate between the upper and
lower limits set by the individuals of absolutely certain genotype (the males).

diamond is shown as representing several different situations along
with their respective degrees of influence upon the phase in the mother
and thereby indirectly upon the risk to the daughter.

   In the first case, the diamond represents a healthy son with marker
allele A1. Since recombination does not occur, he sets the phase in
his mother as A1-normal/A2-disease. The risk for his sister, who also

inherited a maternal A1 allele, is therefore 0%. He has a hypothetical biochemical test result shown in brackets (0.0 to show that he is an obligate noncarrier of the mutation). In the last two cases, the reverse situation is shown, where either an affected son or an obligate carrier daughter inherited the maternal A1 allele. In both of these cases, the risk to daughter II-3 is 100%. In the middle three scenarios, the second child is a daughter with various biochemical test results. When her result is 50%, she is strictly neutral, and we are unable to favor one maternal phase over the other. When her test results are intermediate between 0.00 and 0.50 or intermediate between 0.50 and 1.00, she can be used to make a retrospective assumption about the phase in her mother. The accuracy of his assumption will depend upon how reliable the biochemical test is in discriminating between carriers and noncarriers. Note that the mother and the daughter on the right side have test results indicating likelihoods of 0.8 and 0.2 of being carriers, even though they are both obligate carriers.

8.1.2   Linked Marker, Single Side

In Figure 8.2, we introduced the possibility of recombination by setting $\theta = 0.05$. As in Figure 8.1, II-3 is a female with an unhelpful biochemical test result who wants to know her carrier risk. The diamond in position II-2 again represents one of the scenarios illustrated below the main pedigree. In the first case, II-2 is an unaffected male with the genotype A1. Since he is clinically unaffected, a hypothetical biochemical carrier risk of 0.0 is also shown for him. The fact that he has inherited allele A1 from his mother allows us to retrospectively infer her phase as probably being A1-normal/A2-disease (95% probability). The only time that her phase will be A2-normal/A1-disease instead is when he is a recombinant, which has a probability of 0.05. In the latter two cases, where the mother has passed on A1 and the disease together she has the opposite probabilities of the two phases (A1-d/A2-N = 0.95 and A1-N/A2-d = 0.05). The middle three cases are females with biochemical test results indicating various likelihoods of being carriers. Since their genotypes at the disease locus are not as certain as in the cases where II-2 was a male or an obligate carrier female, it makes sense that their contributions to assigning the probabilities of the two potential phases in their mother should be somewhat less than the upper and lower limits of 0.05 and 0.95 set by the recombination rate applied to male offspring. Females who have a biochemical test result of 0.5 should have no influence whatever on determining the phase of the markers with respect to the disease-causing locus in their mother (in the case of multiple or flanking markers, however,

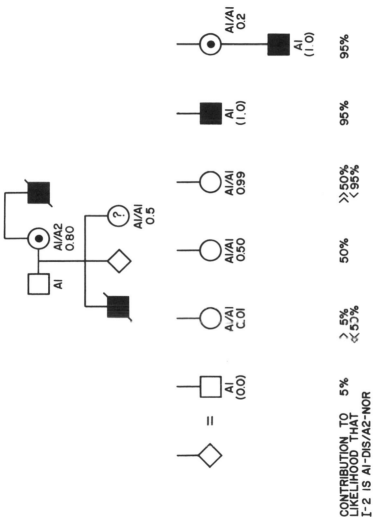

CONTRIBUTION TO   5%   > 5%   50%   >> 50%   95%   95%
LIKELIHOOD THAT   << 50%   << 95%
I-2 IS AI-DIS/A2-NOR

Figure 8.2 This is essentially the same as Fig. 8.1 except that the possibility of recombination has now been introduced ($\phi = 0.05$). The *bottom line* shows the varying degree of influence of the individuals in the center upon the phase of the marker and disease loci in the mother. Since recombination can occur, there is a minimum error of 5%, even when we are absolutely certain of the genotype of the person that we are using to infer phase in the mother.

they can be used to determine the phase of the markers in relation to each other, see section 8.1.3).

To allow us to incorporate females with biochemical test results into phase calculations for their mothers, we need a set of rules. They are as follows:

1. The upper and lower limits will be θ and $1 - \theta$, as in males
2. The midpoint (where a female has a test result of 0.5) will always be neutral, that is, 0.5
3. The scale will be linear, symmetrically compressed between θ and $1 - \theta$ and centered on 0.5

A formula that permits the linear biochemical test results to be compressed into a linear scale bounded by θ and $1 - \theta$ is

$$\text{Value} - \theta + R(0.5 - \theta)/0.5 \tag{8.1}$$

where R = result of biochemical test. If $\theta = 0.05$, this will give results of 0.05, 0.5, and 0.95 when $R = 0$, 0.5, and 1.0, respectively. If $\theta = 0.10$, the same biochemical results would give values of 0.1, 0.5, and 0.9 instead. If a daughter inherits allele A1 from a heterozygous carrier mother and has a biochemical test result that indicates a probability of 0.4 of being a carrier, and if $\theta = 0.10$, the probabilities of the two phases in her mother are A1-d/A2-N (0.42) and A1-N/A2-d (0.58). Tables A.1 and A.2 in the Appendix give the two phase ratios for biochemical test result values between 0.00 and 1.00 at values of θ between 0.00 and 0.10.

If it is necessary to use threshold values instead of a continuous scale of test results (e.g., assuming that $1/3$ of carriers of Duchenne muscular dystrophy have "normal" CK results and $19/20$ noncarriers have "normal" results), then these values can be normalized and the normalized values entered in equation 8.1. The normalized values for $1/3$ and $19/20$ were 0.26 and 0.74 (section 3.1). In Figure 8.3, let us assume that this analysis was performed before the dystrophin gene was cloned and that only one marker at $\theta = 0.10$ was informative.

From formula 8.1, the contribution of II-2 to the determination of the phase in I-2 will be $0.10 + 0.26 (0.4/0.5) = 0.308$ (or conversely, $0.10 + 0.74 (0.4/0.5) = 0.692$, which is the same as $1 - 0.308$). Since II-2 has a normal CK result and also inherited a maternal A1 allele, she should obviously increase the probability that the disease is in coupling with A2 and reduce the probability that it is in coupling with A1 in her mother (Table 8.1).

If II-3 is a carrier, she is phase-known A2-dis-maternal/A1-N-paternal (the father of II-2 must have an A1 allele), which is relevant

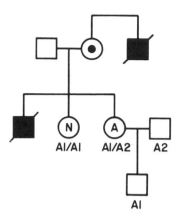

Figure 8.3 A family with a positive family history of Duchenne muscular dystrophy. Marker locus A is linked to the disease at φ = 0.10. The marker genotypes
of the parents can be inferred to be A1 in the father and A1/A2 in the mother.
The influence of II-2 with a maternal A1 allele and a normal creatine kinase (CK)
test result upon the phase in her mother is calculated in Table 8.1. The posterior
probabilities of the phases in the mother are then used to calculate the probability of carrier status in II-3 given her maternal A2 allele, abnormal CK result, and
normal son with an A1 allele (Table 8.2).

Table 8.1   Calculation of the contribution of II-2 in Figure 8.3 to the probability
of each possible phase in her mother

	Phase in I-2	
	A1-dis/A2-N	A1-N/A2-dis
Prior probability	0.5	0.5
Conditional probability		
II-2 has A1 and normal CK†	0.308	0.692
Posterior probability	0.308	0.692

†CK = creatine kinase.

to the conditional probability of having a normal son with the A1 allele
(0.9 under both carrier columns) (Table 8.2). Technically, the DNA
result for II-3 should be part of her prior risk and separate from the
CK result and her son which are conditional risks, but it is easier to
think of the marker genotype as a conditional risk, and it makes no
difference to the outcome.

Table 8.2   Calculation of the risk for II-3 in Figure 8.3

	Phase in I-2			
	A1-dis/A2-N		A1-N/A2-dis	
Posterior probability	0.308		0.692	
II-3 (A1-N/A2-?) =	Carrier	Noncarrier	Carrier	Noncarrier
Conditional probabilities				
maternal A2	0.1	0.9	0.9	0.1
abnormal CK†	0.67	0.05	0.67	0.05
son with A1-N	0.9	1.0	0.9	1.0
Joint probability	0.01857	0.01386	0.37555	0.00346

Carrier total = 0.01857 + 0.37555 = 0.39412 = 95.8%
Noncarrier total − 0.01386 + 0.00346 = 0.01732 = 4.2%

†CK = creatine kinase.

The combination of DNA markers and biochemical test results may potentially be very valuable in the analysis of families where there definitely is or may be a gonadal mosaic carrier of an X-linked disease. As in all cases where a new mutation might be present, it is of considerable importance to try to determine in whom it first occurred. If evidence is available to indicate that a female with a normal (noncarrier) biochemical test result has had more than one affected son, gonadal mosaicism should be carefully considered. If the gene has been cloned, perhaps direct mutation testing will resolve some of the difficult issues such as whether any of her daughters are carriers or the status of a future pregnancy. If the gene has not been cloned, linked markers can indicate inheritance of the at-risk haplotype but will not normally be able to tell if it contains the mutation. Graham et al. (1992) reported a study on a family with a gonadal mosaic for adrenoleukodystrophy, a disease for which the gene has very recently been cloned, but from which there was formerly only a biochemical test that had a 20% false-negative rate in females. It was possible to determine whether the daughters of this female, who had all inherited the at-risk DNA haplotype, were carriers, by using the DNA markers to show that the at-risk haplotypes had subsequently been passed on to normal grandsons. Thus, the normal grandsons retrospectivly diagnosed their mothers as noncarriers of the disease.

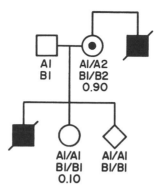

Figure 8.4   A phase-unknown family with a positive family history of an X-linked recessive disease. Marker loci A and B flank the disease locus at $\theta_A = 0.05$ and $\theta_B = 0.10$. The numbers below each female represent the results of a biochemical test used to predict carrier status. Table 8.3 shows the influence that either a normal or an affected male would exert upon the phase in I-2. Table 8.4 shows the influence of daughter II-2 upon the relative probabilities of the four potential phases in I-2. The carrier risk for II-3 is calculated in Table 8.5.

Table 8.3   Calculation of the effect of a normal [or affected] male on the probability of each possible maternal phase in Figure 8.4

A1-N-B1/A2-d-B2 = $(1 - \theta_A) * (1 - \theta_B)$ = 0.95 * 0.90 = 0.855   [0.005]
A1-N-B2/A2-d-B1 = $(1 - \theta_A) * \theta_B$ = 0.95 * 0.10 = 0.095   [0.045]
A2-N-B1/A1-d-B2 = θ_A $* (1 - \theta_B)$ = 0.05 * 0.90 = 0.045   [0.095]
A2-N-B2/A1-d-B1 = θ_A $* \theta_B$ = 0.05 * 0.10 = 0.005   [0.855]

8.1.3   Linked Markers, Flanking

In Figure 8.4, the marker loci A and B flank the disease locus, and there is a biochemical test available that has a continuous scale of linear results. In this particular family, the daughter II-2 has a low risk of being a carrier (10%) according to the biochemical test, and the third pregnancy has inherited the same alleles as II-2. The recombination fractions are $\theta_A = 0.05$ and $\theta_B = 0.10$.

If II-2 were a normal male instead, the calculation of the probabilities of the four potential maternal phases would be straightforward, as shown in Table 8.3. If II-2 were an affected male instead (with the same A1 and B1 alleles), the same numbers would be generated but in reverse order (shown inside the square brackets). It follows from the previous discussion that when II-2 is female, as in the actual example being considered, the probabilities of the maternal phases must fall

Table 8.4   Effect of a daughter, II-2 in Figure 8.4, with different biochemical test results (R) upon the probability of each possible phase in her mother

R	A1-N-B1/ A2-d-B2	A2-N-B1 A1-d-B2	A1-N-B2/ A2-d-B1	A2-N-B2/ A1-d-B1
	Neither Recombinant	A Only Recombinant	B Only Recombinant	Both Recombinant
0.0	0.855	0.045	0.095	0.005
0.1	0.770	0.050	0.090	0.090
0.2	0.685	0.055	0.085	0.175
0.3	0.600	0.060	0.080	0.260
0.4	0.515	0.065	0.075	0.345
0.5	0.430	0.070	0.070	0.430
0.6	0.345	0.075	0.065	0.515
0.7	0.260	0.080	0.060	0.600
0.8	0.175	0.085	0.055	0.685
0.9	0.090	0.090	0.050	0.770
1.0	0.005	0.095	0.045	0.855
	Both Recombinant	B Only Recombinant	A Only Recombinant	Neither Recombinant

within these limits. Table 8.4 gives the probability of each potential maternal phase, given that II-2 has inherited alleles A1 and B1 from her mother, for a series of different biochemical test result values (R).

When the biochemical test results are 0.0 or 1.0 (i.e., she has either 0% risk or 100% risk of being a carrier), the probabilities of each phase are the same as the calculations for males given earlier. When her result is 0.5, there is an equal probability of the disease being associated with A1 or A2 and with B1 or B2 (0.43 + 0.07 for any allele to be in coupling with the disease); however, independent of consideration of her carrier status, she does favor alleles A1 and B1 being in coupling (0.86) rather than in repulsion (0.14). This is the expected result, since they will be in coupling in the mother any time that II-2 is the result of either no crossovers or a double crossover (0.855 + 0.005) and in repulsion any time that II-2 is the result of a single crossover (0.095 + 0.045). If we study just the figures in the left column, at the top, the probability of that maternal phase being correct is 0.855, while, at the bottom, it is 0.005. As the value of R increases toward 0.5, the strength with which the daughter (A1-?-B1) supports that maternal phase (A1-N-B1) being the true one progressively diminishes. Above $R = 0.5$, the daughter starts to count against that phase. At the top and bottom of the column, therefore, it is indicated that her

Table 8.5   Calculation of the carrier risk for II-3 in Figure 8.4

Phase in I-2	Phase	A	B	Total

Probability that II-3 is A1-dis-B1 (carrier)

Phase in I-2	Phase	A	B	Total
A1-Nor-B1/A2-dis-B2 =	0.77 *	0.05 *	0.10 =	0.00385
A1-Nor-B2/A2-dis-B1 =	0.09 *	0.05 *	0.90 =	0.00405
A2-Nor-B1/A1-dis-B2 =	0.05 *	0.95 *	0.10 =	0.00475
A2-Nor-B2/A1-dis-B1 =	0.09 *	0.95 *	0.90 =	0.07695
Carrier total			=	0.08960 = 11.8%

Probability that II-3 is A1-NOR-B1 (noncarrier)

Phase in I-2	Phase	A	B	Total
A1-Nor-B1/A2-dis-B2 =	0.77 *	0.95 *	0.90 =	0.65835
A1-Nor-B2/A2-dis-B1 =	0.09 *	0.95 *	0.10 =	0.00855
A2-Nor-B1/A1-dis-B2 =	0.05 *	0.05 *	0.90 =	0.00225
A2-Nor-B2/A1-dis-B1 =	0.09 *	0.05 *	0.10 =	0.00045
Noncarrier total			=	0.66960 = 88.2%

result progresses from favoring neither marker being recombinant toward favoring both being recombinant, as the result of her biochemical test makes it increasingly likely that she is a carrier. A similar table could be generated for any combination of values of θ by (a) calculating the values at 0.00 and 1.00 (equivalent to those of males), (b) determining the difference between these two values for each phase, and (c) generating the scale for each point 0.## between the limits by adding or subtracting (difference * 0.##).

To return to Figure 8.4, II-2 has a probability of 0.1 of being a carrier, based upon the biochemical test. This gives four numbers for the probabilities of the potential phases in I-2 (0.77, 0.05, 0.09, 0.09). From each of these, the probability that II-3 is a carrier can be calculated given the inheritance of maternal A1 and B1 alleles (Table 8.5). II-3 therefore has a risk of 11.8% of being a carrier of the disease, based upon this information. At some subsequent stage, a biochemical test will be done on II-3, and the pedigree should be reevaluated at that time. One very important point remains: if ever any evidence demonstrates that II-2 is actually a carrier (such as the birth of an affected son), the risk to II-3 is obviously no longer 11.8%, and it must be recalculated (using the phase probabilities from the 1.00 row in Table 8.4 if II-2 is now known to be an obligate carrier).

8.2   Incomplete Penetrance and Age-at-Onset Corrections

Similar logic may be applied when it is necessary to deduce the phase of DNA markers in a parent affected with an autosomal dominant disease. When the offspring of this person have apparently normal phenotypes but may nevertheless be heterozygotes, it is necessary to find a way to incorporate them into risk calculations that allows for the uncertainty of their genotypes at the disease-causing locus.

In the preceding section, where daughters with biochemical test results were used to influence the probability of phase in their mothers, certain rules were developed to ensure that their influence could not exceed that of their brothers and to ensure that when their biochemical test results were noncommittal, their influence on the phase at the disease locus in their mother was neutral (but not their influence on the phase of the DNA markers). In considering nonpenetrance or delayed age at onset, this concept needs modification. Let us consider Huntington disease, where a heterozygote may have a probability anywhere between 0.00 and 1.00 of having symptoms, depending upon whether he or she is a newborn baby or 90 years old. (We are considering delayed age at onset as a model for penetrance as well, since if true penetrance = 0.00, there will be no disease to study, regardless of genotype. A-O will be used as the equivalent of P subject to the caveats discussed in chapter 4.) At birth, heterozygotes for Huntington disease will always have the same phenotype as homozygous normal individuals; at advanced age, the two will always have different phenotypes. The point in the series at which penetrance or age-at-onset corrections should have no influence on parental phase is therefore when P = 0.00 (hypothetical) or A-O = 0.00. The point in the series at which they should exert full influence is when P = 1.00 or A-O = 1.00, since this is when all heterozygotes can be reliably distinguished from homozygotes. The value P = 0.5 or A-O = 0.5 has no particularly special status (as it did when we considered R = 0.5 in biochemical test results on potential carriers of X-linked diseases).

For an affected parent who has informative flanking markers at θ_A = 0.05 and θ_B = 0.10, there are four potential phases (disease-bearing chromosome shown). If that person has an apparently healthy son who inherited an A1-B1 haplotype, as the son ages and progresses through a series of A-O values, he will influence the phase of the loci in his affected parent, as shown in Table 8.6.

When A-O = 0.0, he will influence the phase of the DNA markers only. He inherited the A1-B1 haplotype, which makes it likely that these alleles were in coupling in the parent. Since he has no influence

Table 8.6   Effect of a healthy son with an A1-?-B1 haplotype
at different ages on the probability of the possible parental
phases (only the disease-bearing haplotype is shown)

A-O	A1-D-B1	A2-D-B1	A1-D-B2	A2-D-B2
0.0	0.43	0.07	0.07	0.43
0.1	0.3875	0.0725	0.0675	0.4725
0.2	0.345	0.075	0.065	0.515
0.3	0.3025	0.0775	0.0625	0.5575
0.4	0.26	0.08	0.06	0.6
0.5	0.2175	0.0825	0.0575	0.6425
0.6	0.175	0.085	0.055	0.685
0.7	0.1325	0.0875	0.0525	0.7275
0.8	0.09	0.09	0.05	0.77
0.9	0.0475	0.0925	0.0475	0.8125
1.0	0.005	0.095	0.045	0.855

yet on the disease locus, phases A1-D-B1 and A2-D-B2 are equally
favored (probability of 0.43 each), and phases A1-D-B2 and A2-D-B1
equally disfavored (probability of 0.07 each). When A-O = 1.0, we
know that he is homozygous normal and not heterozygous. Since he
has the A1-n-B1 haplotype, he would need to be a double recombinant
if phase A1-D-B1 was the actual one in his parent. The probability of
his being a double recombinant is 0.005. By similar reasoning, the
probability of his being a single recombinant at locus B (A1-n-B1 from
parental A2-D-B1/A1-n-B2) is 0.095; at locus A, 0.045; and recombinant at neither locus, 0.855.

For other values of θ, a table similar to Table 8.6 could be constructed using the logic given above, or a computer program (written
in BASIC) that generates such data could be used (included in the
Appendix).

Finally, Figure 8.5 shows a graphic representation of the effect of
penetrance or delayed age-at-onset on remaining risk for three values
of θ for a single DNA marker. It is assumed that an individual has been
tested and found to have inherited the high-risk allele in a phase-known
meiosis. When P or A-O = 0.00, the remaining risk = 1 − θ. When
P or A-O = 1.00, the remaining risk is 0.00, since, by definition, all
heterozygotes must be affected. At intermediate values, there is a very
slow reduction in risk until the P or A-O value exceeds approximately
0.8. Beyond that point, it can be seen that small changes in the assumed value of θ make a significant difference to the remaining risk.
(Table A.3 in the Appendix gives the remaining risk for different values

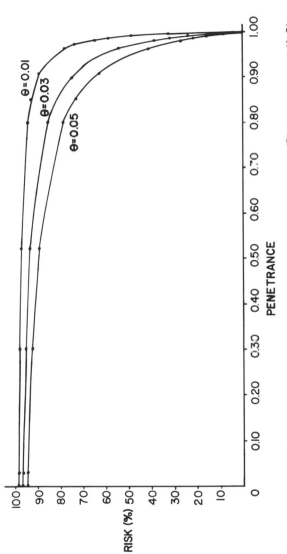

Figure 8.5 A plot of remaining risk of being a heterozygote versus penetrance (P) or age-at-onset (A-O) factor for three different values of θ for an individual who has inherited the high-risk allele from a phase-known meiosis. The risk is initially equal to 1 − θ when P or A-O = 0 and ultimately drops to 0 when P or A-O = 1.0 and it is no longer possible for the person to be a heterozygote. At high values of P or A-O, the effect of using the wrong value of θ becomes very pronounced; at some points, the curves for θ = 0.01 and θ = 0.05 deviate by almost 40%. This graph illustrates that it is potentially a serious error to use the wrong value for θ when phase is being inferred from unaffected individuals.

of P or A-O). For this reason, it was stated in section 6.1 that although the linkage approach gives only an estimate of θ, it is the best available estimate on the currently available data, and it is an error to build in a "margin of safety" by deliberately overestimating the probability of recombination. For several years, this statement had particular relevance to the presymptomatic diagnosis of Huntington disease using linked DNA markers, where the temptation to increase θ "to add a safety factor" may have profoundly influenced the risk in older individuals or the risks for the whole family if phase was inferred from older, currently healthy individuals. Although direct detection of mutations is now possible for Huntington disease and this temptation is no longer relevant, the error should not be repeated for other diseases for which only linked markers are currently available.

Appendix

Decoding Lod Scores

This is the complete listing of the BASIC program to decode lod scores that was discussed in section 6.1. The core part of the program is actually very simple: about half of the code given below is devoted to preventing division by 0 when $\theta = 0.00$ or to avoiding trying to obtain the log of 0. All lines that start with REM are comments that can be omitted.

```
10 CLS
20 REM                  ***** PROGRAM TO DECODE LOD SCORES  *****
30 REM                  *****            BY               *****
40 REM                  *****   PETER J. BRIDGE, Ph.D.    *****
50 PRINT
60 REM Remember that all aspects of this program assume that the data were
70 REM originally obtained from phase-known meioses only.
80 PRINT"ENTER THE VALUE OF Zmax TO BE DECODED":INPUT A
90 IF A<0 THEN PRINT"POSITIVE VALUES ONLY.    THIS DECODES Zmax NOT Z":GOTO 50
100 PRINT
110 REM To type θ hold down ALT while you type 233 on the numerical keypad.
120 PRINT"ENTER THE θmax FOR THAT VALUE OF Zmax":INPUT B
130 IF B<0 THEN PRINT"DON'T BE SILLY. θ CANNOT BE NEGATIVE":GOTO 100
140 IF B>.49 THEN PRINT"θmax MUST BE LESS THAN 0.49":GOTO 100
150 PRINT
160 LET C = 1-B:LET D = B*100:LET E = C*100:LET N = 2.3025851#
170 IF B = 0 THEN GOTO 200
```

180 LET F = LOG(B)

190 GOTO 210

200 LET F = 0

210 LET G = (100*LOG(2) + E*LOG(C) + D*F)/N

220 LET RATIO = A/G

230 LET MEIOSES = RATIO*100

240 LET RECS = RATIO*D

250 IF B = 0 THEN LET T = 0:GOTO 320

260 FOR R = .001 TO B STEP .001

270 LET S = (MEIOSES*LOG(2) + (MEIOSES-RECS)*LOG(1-R) + RECS*LOG(R))/N

280 IF S>G*RATIO-1 THEN GOTO 330

290 LET T = R

300 NEXT R

310 GOTO 330

320 LET X = .001:GOTO 340

330 LET X = B

340 FOR U = X TO .499 STEP .001

350 LET V = (MEIOSES*LOG(2) + (MEIOSES-RECS)*LOG(1-U) + RECS*LOG(U))/N

360 IF V<G*RATIO-1 THEN GOTO 390

370 LET W = U

380 NEXT U

390 CLS

400 PRINT"FIRST ESTIMATE IS "RECS" RECOMBINANTS OUT OF "MEIOSES

410 PRINT"PHASE-KNOWN MEIOSES WOULD GIVE Zmax = "G*RATIO" AT θmax = "B

420 PRINT"CONFIDENCE INTERVALS FOR θ WOULD BE APPROXIMATELY "T" TO "W:PRINT

430 PRINT"RANGE OF INTEGRAL NUMBERS AROUND ESTIMATE − TAKE YOUR PICK":PRINT

440 PRINT"RECOMBINANTS","MEIOSES","Zmax","θmax":PRINT

450 LET A1 = INT(RECS):LET A2 = INT(MEIOSES)

460 IF A1<2 THEN GOTO 560

470 IF A2<2 THEN GOTO 560

480 FOR I = A1-1 TO A1 + 1

490 FOR J = A2-1 TO A2 + 2

500 LET K = I/J:LET L = 1-K:LET M = J-I

510 LET Z = (J*LOG(2) + M*LOG(L) + I*LOG(K))/N

520 PRINT I,J,Z,K

530 NEXT J

540 NEXT I

550 GOTO 710

560 FOR I = 0 TO 2

570 FOR J = A2-1 TO A2 + 2

580 IF I>J THEN GOTO 690

590 REM Can't have more recombinants than children

600 IF J<1 THEN LET Z = 0:GOTO 680

610 LET K = I/J:LET L = 1-K:LET M = J-I

620 IF I = 0 THEN LET P = 0:GOTO 640

630 LET P = LOG(K)

640 IF L = 0 THEN LET Q = 0:GOTO 660

650 LET Q = LOG(L)

660 LET Z = (J*LOG(2) + M*Q + I*P)/N

670 IF K> = .5 THEN LET K = .5:LET Z = 0

680 PRINT I,J,Z,K

690 NEXT J

700 NEXT I

710 LET K = 0

720 PRINT"ENTER 1 TO CONTINUE, 2 TO QUIT OR 3 TO EXIT TO DOS":INPUT Y

730 ON Y GOTO 10,740,750

740 END

750 SYSTEM

For very slow computers, the following modifications should speed up the analysis.

260 FOR R = .01 TO B STEP .01

320 LET X = .01:GOTO 340

340 FOR U = X TO .49 STEP .01

Pascal's Triangle and the Binomial Expansion

$$
\begin{array}{ccccccc}
 & & & 1 & 1 & & \\
 & & 1 & 2 & 1 & & \\
 & 1 & 3 & 3 & 1 & & \\
 1 & 4 & 6 & 4 & 1 & & \\
1 & 5 & 10 & 10 & 5 & 1 & \\
1 & 6 & 15 & 20 & 15 & 6 & 1
\end{array}
$$

$$
\begin{array}{ccccccc}
 & & & p & q & & \\
 & & p^2 & pq & q^2 & & \\
 & p^3 & p^2q & pq^2 & q^3 & & \\
 p^4 & p^3q & p^2q^2 & pq^3 & q^4 & & \\
p^5 & p^4q & p^3q^2 & p^2q^3 & pq^4 & q^5 & \\
p^6 & p^5q & p^4q^2 & p^3q^3 & p^2q^4 & pq^5 & q^6
\end{array}
$$

In Pascal's triangle, each number is generated by adding together the two numbers immediately above it. The numbers in this pyramid form the coefficients that precede each of the terms of $p^N q^N$; thus the expansion of the binomial expression $(p + q)^4$ is $p^4 + 4p^3q + 6p^2q^2 + 4pq^3 + q^4$. The binomial theorem is used in human genetics to determine the probability of a series of events, each step of which has two alternative outcomes, the sum of the frequencies of which is 1.0. For instance, the probability of having precisely 4 boys and 1 girl out of 5 children is $5p^4q$ where $p = q = 0.5$ ($= 5/32$ or 0.15625).

If parents who are carriers of an autosomal recessive disease, have three children, the following patterns can be predicted (p = normal $= 0.75$; q = affected $= 0.25$).

3 normal	$= p^3$	$= (0.75)^3$		$= 27/64$	$= 0.421875$
2 normal, 1 affected	$= 3p^2q$	$= 3(0.75)^2(0.25)$		$= 27/64$	$= 0.421875$
1 normal, 2 affected	$= 3pq^2$	$= 3(0.75)(0.25)^2$		$= 9/64$	$= 0.140625$
3 affected	$= q^3$	$= (0.25)^3$		$- 1/64$	$- 0.015625$

Program to Generate Phase Values for Flanking Markers and Reduced Penetrance or Delayed Age at Onset

```
10 CLS
20 REM Flanking markers with penetrance or age-at-onset
30 REM Peter J. Bridge, Ph.D., FCCMG, FACMG
40 PRINT"ENTER 1 FOR SINGLE CASE, 2 FOR TABLE OF VALUES, 3 TO QUIT, 4 FOR
DOS":INPUT Z1
50 ON Z1 GOTO 60,60,670,680
60 PRINT
70 PRINT"INPUT THETA-A, THETA-B"
80 PRINT"THETA-B SHOULD NOT BE SMALLER THAN THETA-A":INPUT A,B
90 IF A>B GOTO 70
100 LET C = 1-A
110 LET D = 1-B
120 LET P1 = C*D
130 LET P2 = A*D
140 LET P3 = B*C
150 LET P4 = A*B
160 PRINT
170 ON Z1 GOTO 180,390,670
```

```
180 PRINT"A-COUPLING/B-COUPLING   = "P1
190 PRINT"A-REPULSION/B-COUPLING   = "P2
200 PRINT"A-COUPLING/B-REPULSION   = "P3
210 PRINT"A-REPULSION/B-REPULSION  = "P4
220 PRINT
230 ON Z1 GOTO 240,390,670
240 PRINT"INPUT PENETRANCE VALUE":INPUT E
250 LET F  =  (C-B)/2
260 LET G  =  (B-A)/2
270 LET H  =  (P1 + P4)/2-E*F
280 LET I  =  (P2 + P3)/2 + E*G
290 LET J  =  (P2 + P3)/2-E*G
300 LET K  =  (P4 + P1)/2 + E*F
310 PRINT
320 PRINT"Ac-n-Bc","Ar-n-Bc","Ac-n-Br","Ar-n-Br","r = in repulsion"
330 PRINT"  or","  or","  or","  or"
340 PRINT"Ar-D-Br","Ac-D-Br","Ar-D-Bc","Ac-D-Bc","c = in coupling"
350 PRINT
360 PRINT H,I,J,K
370 PRINT
380 GOTO 40
390 PRINT"ENTER THE RANGE FOR PENETRANCE"
400 PRINT"ENTER AS LOW,HIGH,INCREMENT (EG, 0,.5,.05)":INPUT E1,E2,E3
410 PRINT
420 PRINT"RESULTS ON SCREEN = 1, ON PRINTER = 2, ON DISK = 3":INPUT Z3
430 ON Z3 GOTO 460,460,440
440 PRINT"ENTER NAME FOR FILE":INPUT FILENAME$
450 OPEN FILENAME$ FOR OUTPUT AS #1
460 LET F = (C-B)/2
470 LET G = (B-A)/2
480 PRINT"Ac-n-Bc","Ar-n-Bc","Ac-n-Br","Ar-n-Br","r = in repulsion"
490 PRINT"  or","  or","  or","  or"
500 PRINT"Ar-D-Br","Ac-D-Br","Ar-D-Bc","Ac-D-Bc","c = in coupling"
510 PRINT
520 FOR Z2 = E1 TO E2 STEP E3
530 LET H  =  (P1 + P4)/2-Z2*F
540 LET I  =  (P2 + P3)/2 + Z2*G
```

```
550 LET J  =  (P2 + P3)/2-Z2*G
560 LET K  =  (P4 + P1)/2 + Z2*F
570 ON Z3 GOTO 580,600,620
580 PRINT H,I,J,K,"PEN = "Z2
590 GOTO 630
600 LPRINT H,I,J,K,"PEN = "Z2
610 GOTO 630
620 WRITE #1,Z2,H,I,J,K
630 NEXT Z2
640 IF Z3 = 3 THEN CLOSE #1
650 PRINT
660 GOTO 40
670 END
680 SYSTEM
```

Table A.1   Non-DNA Test Result (R) versus Phase Ratios for θ = 0.00 to 0.05

	θ					
R	0.00	0.01	0.02	0.03	0.04	0.05
0.00	.0000, 1.000	.0100, .9900	.0200, .9800	.0300, .9700	.0400, .9600	.0500, .9500
0.01	.0100, .9900	.0198, .9802	.0296, .9704	.0394, .9606	.0492, .9508	.0590, .9410
0.02	.0200, .9800	.0296, .9704	.0392, .9608	.0488, .9512	.0584, .9416	.0680, .9320
0.03	.0300, .9700	.0394, .9606	.0488, .9512	.0582, .9418	.0676, .9324	.0770, .9230
0.04	.0400, .9600	.0492, .9508	.0584, .9416	.0676, .9324	.0768, .9232	.0860, .9140
0.05	.0500, .9500	.0590, .9410	.0680, .9320	.0770, .9230	.0860, .9140	.0950, .9050
0.06	.0600, .9400	.0688, .9312	.0776, .9224	.0864, .9136	.0952, .9048	.1040, .8960
0.07	.0700, .9300	.0786, .9214	.0872, .9128	.0958, .9042	.1044, .8956	.1130, .8870
0.08	.0800, .9200	.0884, .9116	.0968, .9032	.1052, .8948	.1136, .8864	.1220, .8780
0.09	.0900, .9100	.0982, .9018	.1064, .8936	.1146, .8854	.1228, .8772	.1310, .8690
0.10	.1000, .9000	.1080, .8920	.1160, .8840	.1240, .8760	.1320, .8680	.1400, .8600
0.11	.1100, .8900	.1178, .8822	.1256, .8744	.1334, .8666	.1412, .8588	.1490, .8510
0.12	.1200, .8800	.1276, .8724	.1352, .8648	.1428, .8572	.1504, .8496	.1580, .8420
0.13	.1300, .8700	.1374, .8626	.1448, .8552	.1522, .8478	.1596, .8404	.1670, .8330
0.14	.1400, .8600	.1472, .8528	.1544, .8456	.1616, .8384	.1688, .8312	.1760, .8240
0.15	.1500, .8500	.1570, .8430	.1640, .8360	.1710, .8290	.1780, .8220	.1850, .8150
0.16	.1600, .8400	.1668, .8332	.1736, .8264	.1804, .8196	.1872, .8128	.1940, .8060
0.17	.1700, .8300	.1766, .8234	.1832, .8168	.1898, .8102	.1964, .8036	.2030, .7970
0.18	.1800, .8200	.1864, .8136	.1928, .8072	.1992, .8008	.2056, .7944	.2120, .7880
0.19	.1900, .8100	.1962, .8038	.2024, .7976	.2086, .7914	.2148, .7852	.2210, .7790
0.20	.2000, .8000	.2060, .7940	.2120, .7880	.2180, .7820	.2240, .7760	.2300, .7700
0.21	.2100, .7900	.2158, .7842	.2216, .7784	.2274, .7726	.2332, .7668	.2390, .7610
0.22	.2200, .7800	.2256, .7744	.2312, .7688	.2368, .7632	.2424, .7576	.2480, .7520

Table A.1 (Continued)

			θ			
R	0.00	0.01	0.02	0.03	0.04	0.05
0.23	.2300, .7700	.2354, .7646	.2408, .7592	.2462, .7538	.2516, .7484	.2570, .7430
0.24	.2400, .7600	.2452, .7548	.2504, .7496	.2556, .7444	.2608, .7392	.2660, .7340
0.25	.2500, .7500	.2550, .7450	.2600, .7400	.2650, .7350	.2700, .7300	.2750, .7250
0.26	.2600, .7400	.2648, .7352	.2696, .7304	.2744, .7256	.2792, .7208	.2840, .7160
0.27	.2700, .7300	.2746, .7254	.2792, .7208	.2838, .7162	.2884, .7116	.2930, .7070
0.28	.2800, .7200	.2844, .7156	.2888, .7112	.2932, .7068	.2976, .7024	.3020, .6980
0.29	.2900, .7100	.2942, .7058	.2984, .7016	.3026, .6974	.3068, .6932	.3110, .6890
0.30	.3000, .7000	.3040, .6960	.3080, .6920	.3120, .6880	.3160, .6840	.3200, .6800
0.31	.3100, .6900	.3138, .6862	.3176, .6824	.3214, .6786	.3252, .6748	.3290, .6710
0.32	.3200, .6800	.3236, .6764	.3272, .6728	.3308, .6692	.3344, .6656	.3380, .6620
0.33	.3300, .6700	.3334, .6666	.3368, .6632	.3402, .6598	.3436, .6564	.3470, .6530
0.34	.3400, .6600	.3432, .6568	.3464, .6536	.3496, .6504	.3528, .6472	.3560, .6440
0.35	.3500, .6500	.3530, .6470	.3560, .6440	.3590, .6410	.3620, .6380	.3650, .6350
0.36	.3600, .6400	.3628, .6372	.3656, .6344	.3684, .6316	.3712, .6288	.3740, .6260
0.37	.3700, .6300	.3726, .6274	.3752, .6248	.3778, .6222	.3804, .6196	.3830, .6170
0.38	.3800, .6200	.3824, .6176	.3848, .6152	.3872, .6128	.3896, .6104	.3920, .6080
0.39	.3900, .6100	.3922, .6078	.3944, .6056	.3966, .6034	.3988, .6012	.4010, .5990
0.40	.4000, .6000	.4020, .5980	.4040, .5960	.4060, .5940	.4080, .5920	.4100, .5900
0.41	.4100, .5900	.4118, .5882	.4136, .5864	.4154, .5846	.4172, .5828	.4190, .5810
0.42	.4200, .5800	.4216, .5784	.4232, .5768	.4248, .5752	.4264, .5736	.4280, .5720
0.43	.4300, .5700	.4314, .5686	.4328, .5672	.4342, .5658	.4356, .5644	.4370, .5630
0.44	.4400, .5600	.4412, .5588	.4424, .5576	.4436, .5564	.4448, .5552	.4460, .5540
0.45	.4500, .5500	.4510, .5490	.4520, .5480	.4530, .5470	.4540, .5460	.4550, .5450
0.46	.4600, .5400	.4608, .5392	.4616, .5384	.4624, .5376	.4632, .5368	.4640, .5360
0.47	.4700, .5300	.4706, .5294	.4712, .5288	.4718, .5282	.4724, .5276	.4730, .5270
0.48	.4800, .5200	.4804, .5196	.4808, .5192	.4812, .5188	.4816, .5184	.4820, .5180
0.49	.4900, .5100	.4902, .5098	.4904, .5096	.4906, .5094	.4908, .5092	.4910, .5090
0.50	.5000, .5000	.5000, .5000	.5000, .5000	.5000, .5000	.5000, .5000	.5000, .5000
0.51	.5100, .4900	.5098, .4902	.5096, .4904	.5094, .4906	.5092, .4908	.5090, .4910
0.52	.5200, .4800	.5196, .4804	.5192, .4808	.5188, .4812	.5184, .4816	.5180, .4820
0.53	.5300, .4700	.5294, .4706	.5288, .4712	.5282, .4718	.5276, .4724	.5270, .4730
0.54	.5400, .4600	.5392, .4608	.5384, .4616	.5376, .4624	.5368, .4632	.5360, .4640
0.55	.5500, .4500	.5490, .4510	.5480, .4520	.5470, .4530	.5460, .4540	.5450, .4550
0.56	.5600, .4400	.5588, .4412	.5576, .4424	.5564, .4436	.5552, .4448	.5540, .4460
0.57	.5700, .4300	.5686, .4314	.5672, .4328	.5658, .4342	.5644, .4356	.5630, .4370
0.58	.5800, .4200	.5784, .4216	.5768, .4232	.5752, .4248	.5736, .4264	.5720, .4280
0.59	.5900, .4100	.5882, .4118	.5864, .4136	.5846, .4154	.5828, .4172	.5810, .4190
0.60	.6000, .4000	.5980, .4020	.5960, .4040	.5940, .4060	.5920, .4080	.5900, .4100
0.61	.6100, .3900	.6078, .3922	.6056, .3944	.6034, .3966	.6012, .3988	.5990, .4010
0.62	.6200, .3800	.6176, .3824	.6152, .3848	.6128, .3872	.6104, .3896	.6080, .3920
0.63	.6300, .3700	.6274, .3726	.6248, .3752	.6222, .3778	.6196, .3804	.6170, .3830
0.64	.6400, .3600	.6372, .3628	.6344, .3656	.6316, .3684	.6288, .3712	.6260, .3740
0.65	.6500, .3500	.6470, .3530	.6440, .3560	.6410, .3590	.6380, .3620	.6350, .3650
0.66	.6600, .3400	.6568, .3432	.6536, .3464	.6504, .3496	.6472, .3528	.6440, .3560

Table A.1 (Continued)

R	0.00	0.01	0.02	0.03	0.04	0.05
				θ		
0.67	.6700, .3300	.6666, .3334	.6632, .3368	.6598, .3402	.6564, .3436	.6530, .3470
0.68	.6800, .3200	.6764, .3236	.6728, .3272	.6692, .3308	.6656, .3344	.6620, .3380
0.69	.6900, .3100	.6862, .3138	.6824, .3176	.6786, .3214	.6748, .3252	.6710, .3290
0.70	.7000, .3000	.6960, .3040	.6920, .3080	.6880, .3120	.6840, .3160	.6800, .3200
0.71	.7100, .2900	.7058, .2942	.7016, .2984	.6974, .3026	.6932, .3068	.6890, .3110
0.72	.7200, .2800	.7156, .2844	.7112, .2888	.7068, .2932	.7024, .2976	.6980, .3020
0.73	.7300, .2700	.7254, .2746	.7208, .2792	.7162, .2838	.7116, .2884	.7070, .2930
0.74	.7400, .2600	.7352, .2648	.7304, .2696	.7256, .2744	.7208, .2792	.7160, .2840
0.75	.7500, .2500	.7450, .2550	.7400, .2600	.7350, .2650	.7300, .2700	.7250, .2750
0.76	.7600, .2400	.7548, .2452	.7496, .2504	.7444, .2556	.7392, .2608	.7340, .2660
0.77	.7700, .2300	.7646, .2354	.7592, .2408	.7538, .2462	.7484, .2516	.7430, .2570
0.78	.7800, .2200	.7744, .2256	.7688, .2312	.7632, .2368	.7576, .2424	.7520, .2480
0.79	.7900, .2100	.7842, .2158	.7784, .2216	.7726, .2274	.7668, .2332	.7610, .2390
0.80	.8000, .2000	.7940, .2060	.7880, .2120	.7820, .2180	.7760, .2240	.7700, .2300
0.81	.8100, .1900	.8038, .1962	.7976, .2024	.7914, .2086	.7852, .2148	.7790, .2210
0.82	.8200, .1800	.8136, .1864	.8072, .1928	.8008, .1992	.7944, .2056	.7880, .2120
0.83	.8300, .1700	.8234, .1766	.8168, .1832	.8102, .1898	.8036, .1964	.7970, .2030
0.84	.8400, .1600	.8332, .1668	.8264, .1736	.8196, .1804	.8128, .1872	.8060, .1940
0.85	.8500, .1500	.8430, .1570	.8360, .1640	.8290, .1710	.8220, .1780	.8150, .1850
0.86	.8600, .1400	.8528, .1472	.8456, .1544	.8384, .1616	.8312, .1688	.8240, .1760
0.87	.8700, .1300	.8626, .1374	.8552, .1448	.8478, .1522	.8404, .1596	.8330, .1670
0.88	.8800, .1200	.8724, .1276	.8648, .1352	.8572, .1428	.8496, .1504	.8420, .1580
0.89	.8900, .1100	.8822, .1178	.8744, .1256	.8666, .1334	.8588, .1412	.8510, .1490
0.90	.9000, .1000	.8920, .1080	.8840, .1160	.8760, .1240	.8680, .1320	.8600, .1400
0.91	.9100, .0900	.9018, .0982	.8936, .1064	.8854, .1146	.8772, .1228	.8690, .1310
0.92	.9200, .0800	.9116, .0884	.9032, .0968	.8948, .1052	.8864, .1136	.8780, .1220
0.93	.9300, .0700	.9214, .0786	.9128, .0872	.9042, .0958	.8956, .1044	.8870, .1130
0.94	.9400, .0600	.9312, .0688	.9224, .0776	.9136, .0864	.9048, .0952	.8960, .1040
0.95	.9500, .0500	.9410, .0590	.9320, .0680	.9230, .0770	.9140, .0860	.9050, .0950
0.96	.9600, .0400	.9508, .0492	.9416, .0584	.9324, .0676	.9232, .0768	.9140, .0860
0.97	.9700, .0300	.9606, .0394	.9512, .0488	.9418, .0582	.9324, .0676	.9230, .0770
0.98	.9800, .0200	.9704, .0296	.9608, .0392	.9512, .0488	.9416, .0584	.9320, .0680
0.99	.9900, .0100	.9802, .0198	.9704, .0296	.9606, .0394	.9508, .0492	.9410, .0590
1.00	1.000, .0000	.9900, .0100	.9800, .0200	.9700, .0300	.9600, .0400	.9500, .0500

Table A.2   Non-DNA Test Result (*R*) versus Phase Ratios for θ = 0.06 to 0.10

			θ		
R	0.06	0.07	0.08	0.09	0.10
0.00	.0600, .9400	.0700, .9300	.0800, .9200	.0900, .9100	.1000, .9000
0.01	.0688, .9312	.0786, .9214	.0884, .9116	.0982, .9018	.1080, .8920
0.02	.0776, .9224	.0872, .9128	.0968, .9032	.1064, .8936	.1160, .8840
0.03	.0864, .9136	.0958, .9042	.1052, .8948	.1146, .8854	.1240, .8760
0.04	.0952, .9048	.1044, .8956	.1136, .8864	.1228, .8772	.1320, .8680
0.05	.1040, .8960	.1130, .8870	.1220, .8780	.1310, .8690	.1400, .8600
0.06	.1128, .8872	.1216, .8784	.1304, .8696	.1392, .8608	.1480, .8520
0.07	.1216, .8784	.1302, .8698	.1388, .8612	.1474, .8526	.1560, .8440
0.08	.1304, .8696	.1388, .8612	.1472, .8528	.1556, .8444	.1640, .8360
0.09	.1392, .8608	.1474, .8526	.1556, .8444	.1638, .8362	.1720, .8280
0.10	.1480, .8520	.1560, .8440	.1640, .8360	.1720, .8280	.1800, .8200
0.11	.1568, .8432	.1646, .8354	.1724, .8276	.1802, .8198	.1880, .8120
0.12	.1656, .8344	.1732, .8268	.1808, .8192	.1884, .8116	.1960, .8040
0.13	.1744, .8256	.1818, .8182	.1892, .8108	.1966, .8034	.2040, .7960
0.14	.1832, .8168	.1904, .8096	.1976, .8024	.2048, .7952	.2120, .7880
0.15	.1920, .8080	.1990, .8010	.2060, .7940	.2130, .7870	.2200, .7800
0.16	.2008, .7992	.2076, .7924	.2144, .7856	.2212, .7788	.2280, .7720
0.17	.2096, .7904	.2162, .7838	.2228, .7772	.2294, .7706	.2360, .7640
0.18	.2184, .7816	.2248, .7752	.2312, .7688	.2376, .7624	.2440, .7560
0.19	.2272, .7728	.2334, .7666	.2396, .7604	.2458, .7542	.2520, .7480
0.20	.2360, .7640	.2420, .7580	.2480, .7520	.2540, .7460	.2600, .7400
0.21	.2448, .7552	.2506, .7494	.2564, .7436	.2600, .7378	.2680, .7320
0.22	.2536, .7464	.2592, .7408	.2648, .7352	.2704, .7296	.2760, .7240
0.23	.2624, .7376	.2678, .7322	.2732, .7268	.2786, .7214	.2840, .7160
0.24	.2712, .7288	.2764, .7236	.2816, .7184	.2868, .7132	.2920, .7080
0.25	.2800, .7200	.2850, .7150	.2900, .7100	.2950, .7050	.3000, .7000
0.26	.2888, .7112	.2936, .7064	.2984, .7016	.3032, .6968	.3080, .6920
0.27	.2976, .7024	.3022, .6978	.3068, .6932	.3114, .6886	.3160, .6840
0.28	.3064, .6936	.3108, .6892	.3152, .6848	.3196, .6804	.3240, .6760
0.29	.3152, .6848	.3194, .6806	.3236, .6764	.3278, .6722	.3320, .6680
0.30	.3240, .6760	.3280, .6720	.3320, .6680	.3360, .6640	.3400, .6600
0.31	.3328, .6672	.3366, .6634	.3404, .6596	.3442, .6558	.3480, .6520
0.32	.3416, .6584	.3452, .6548	.3488, .6512	.3524, .6476	.3560, .6440
0.33	.3504, .6496	.3538, .6462	.3572, .6428	.3606, .6394	.3640, .6360
0.34	.3592, .6408	.3624, .6376	.3656, .6344	.3688, .6312	.3720, .6280
0.35	.3680, .6320	.3710, .6290	.3740, .6260	.3770, .6230	.3800, .6200
0.36	.3768, .6232	.3796, .6204	.3824, .6176	.3852, .6148	.3880, .6120
0.37	.3856, .6144	.3882, .6118	.3908, .6092	.3934, .6066	.3960, .6040
0.38	.3944, .6056	.3968, .6032	.3992, .6008	.4016, .5984	.4040, .5960
0.39	.4032, .5968	.4054, .5946	.4076, .5924	.4098, .5902	.4120, .5880
0.40	.4120, .5880	.4140, .5860	.4160, .5840	.4180, .5820	.4200, .5800
0.41	.4208, .5792	.4226, .5774	.4244, .5756	.4262, .5738	.4280, .5720
0.42	.4296, .5704	.4312, .5688	.4328, .5672	.4344, .5656	.4360, .5640
0.43	.4384, .5616	.4398, .5602	.4412, .5588	.4426, .5574	.4440, .5560

Table A.2 (Continued)

R	0.06	0.07	θ 0.08	0.09	0.10
0.44	.4472, .5528	.4484, .5516	.4496, .5504	.4508, .5492	.4520, .5480
0.45	.4560, .5440	.4570, .5430	.4580, .5420	.4590, .5410	.4600, .5400
0.46	.4648, .5352	.4656, .5344	.4664, .5336	.4672, .5328	.4680, .5320
0.47	.4736, .5264	.4742, .5258	.4748, .5252	.4754, .5246	.4760, .5240
0.48	.4824, .5176	.4828, .5172	.4832, .5168	.4836, .5164	.4840, .5160
0.49	.4912, .5088	.4914, .5086	.4916, .5084	.4918, .5082	.4920, .5080
0.50	.5000, .5000	.5000, .5000	.5000, .5000	.5000, .5000	.5000, .5000
0.51	.5088, .4912	.5086, .4914	.5084, .4916	.5082, .4918	.5080, .4920
0.52	.5176, .4824	.5172, .4828	.5168, .4832	.5164, .4836	.5160, .4840
0.53	.5264, .4736	.5258, .4742	.5252, .4748	.5246, .4754	.5240, .4760
0.54	.5352, .4648	.5344, .4656	.5336, .4664	.5328, .4672	.5320, .4680
0.55	.5440, .4560	.5430, .4570	.5420, .4580	.5410, .4590	.5400, .4600
0.56	.5528, .4472	.5516, .4484	.5504, .4496	.5492, .4508	.5480, .4520
0.57	.5616, .4384	.5602, .4398	.5588, .4412	.5574, .4426	.5560, .4440
0.58	.5704, .4296	.5688, .4312	.5672, .4328	.5656, .4344	.5640, .4360
0.59	.5792, .4208	.5774, .4226	.5756, .4244	.5738, .4262	.5720, .4280
0.60	.5880, .4120	.5860, .4140	.5840, .4160	.5820, .4180	.5800, .4200
0.61	.5968, .4032	.5946, .4054	.5924, .4076	.5902, .4098	.5880, .4120
0.62	.6056, .3944	.6032, .3968	.6008, .3992	.5984, .4016	.5960, .4040
0.63	.6144, .3856	.6118, .3882	.6092, .3908	.6066, .3934	.6040, .3960
0.64	.6232, .3768	.6204, .3796	.6176, .3824	.6148, .3852	.6120, .3880
0.65	.6320, .3680	.6290, .3710	.6260, .3740	.6230, .3770	.6200, .3800
0.66	.6408, .3592	.6376, .3624	.6344, .3656	.6312, .3688	.6280, .3720
0.67	.6496, .3504	.6462, .3538	.6428, .3572	.6394, .3606	.6360, .3640
0.68	.6584, .3416	.6548, .3452	.6512, .3488	.6476, .3524	.6440, .3560
0.69	.6672, .3328	.6634, .3366	.6596, .3404	.6558, .3442	.6520, .3480
0.70	.6760, .3240	.6720, .3280	.6680, .3320	.6640, .3360	.6600, .3400
0.71	.6848, .3152	.6806, .3194	.6764, .3236	.6722, .3278	.6680, .3320
0.72	.6936, .3064	.6892, .3108	.6848, .3152	.6804, .3196	.6760, .3240
0.73	.7024, .2976	.6988, .3022	.6932, .3068	.6886, .3114	.6840, .3160
0.74	.7112, .2888	.7064, .2936	.7016, .2984	.6968, .3032	.6920, .3080
0.75	.7200, .2800	.7150, .2850	.7100, .2900	.7050, .2950	.7000, .3000
0.76	.7288, .2712	.7236, .2764	.7184, .2816	.7132, .2868	.7080, .2920
0.77	.7376, .2624	.7322, .2678	.7268, .2732	.7214, .2786	.7160, .2840
0.78	.7464, .2536	.7408, .2592	.7352, .2648	.7296, .2704	.7240, .2760
0.79	.7552, .2448	.7494, .2506	.7436, .2564	.7378, .2622	.7320, .2680
0.80	.7640, .2360	.7580, .2420	.7520, .2480	.7460, .2540	.7400, .2600
0.81	.7728, .2272	.7666, .2334	.7604, .2396	.7542, .2458	.7480, .2520
0.82	.7816, .2184	.7752, .2248	.7688, .2312	.7624, .2376	.7560, .2440
0.83	.7904, .2096	.7838, .2162	.7772, .2228	.7706, .2294	.7640, .2360
0.84	.7992, .2008	.7924, .2076	.7856, .2144	.7788, .2212	.7720, .2280
0.85	.8080, .1920	.8010, .1990	.7940, .2060	.7870, .2130	.7800, .2200
0.86	.8168, .1832	.8096, .1904	.8024, .1976	.7952, .2048	.7880, .2120
0.87	.8256, .1744	.8182, .1818	.8108, .1892	.8034, .1966	.7960, .2040

Table A.2 (Continued)

			θ		
R	0.06	0.07	0.08	0.09	0.10
0.88	.8344, .1656	.8268, .1732	.8192, .1808	.8116, .1884	.8040, .1960
0.89	.8432, .1568	.8354, .1646	.8276, .1724	.8198, .1802	.8120, .1880
0.90	.8520, .1480	.8405, .1560	.8360, .1640	.8280, .1720	.8200, .1800
0.91	.8608, .1392	.8526, .1474	.8444, .1556	.8362, .1638	.8280, .1720
0.92	.8696, .1304	.8612, .1388	.8528, .1472	.8444, .1556	.8360, .1640
0.93	.8784, .1216	.8698, .1302	.8612, .1388	.8526, .1474	.8440, .1560
0.94	.8872, .1128	.8784, .1216	.8696, .1304	.8608, .1392	.8520, .1480
0.95	.8960, .1040	.8870, .1130	.8780, .1220	.8690, .1310	.8600, .1400
0.96	.9048, .0952	.8956, .1044	.8864, .1136	.8772, .1228	.8680, .1320
0.97	.9136, .0864	.9042, .0958	.8948, .1052	.8854, .1146	.8760, .1240
0.98	.9224, .0776	.9128, .0872	.9032, .0968	.8936, .1064	.8840, .1160
0.99	.9312, .0688	.9214, .0786	.9116, .0884	.9018, .0982	.8920, .1080
1.00	.9400, .0600	.9300, .0700	.9200, .0800	.9100, .0900	.9000, .1000

Table A.3   Remaining Risk at Various Values of θ and Penetrance (P)

			θ		
P	0.01	0.02	0.03	0.04	0.05	0.06
0.00	.9900000	.9800000	.9700000	.9600000	.9500000	.9400000
0.01	.9899000	.9798021	.9697062	.9596122	.9495204	.9394306
0.02	.9897980	.9796002	.9694065	.9592169	.9490316	.9388504
0.03	.9896939	.9793942	.9691009	.9588139	.9485332	.9382589
0.04	.9895877	.9791841	.9687891	.9584026	.9480249	.9376559
0.05	.9894792	.9789695	.9684709	.9579832	.9475066	.9370409
0.06	.9893685	.9787505	.9681461	.9575552	.9469778	.9364137
0.07	.9892554	.9785269	.9678146	.9571183	.9464381	.9357739
0.08	.9891399	.9782986	.9674762	.9566724	.9458874	.9351211
0.09	.9890218	.9780654	.9671306	.9562172	.9453253	.9344549
0.10	.9889012	.9778271	.9667774	.9557522	.9447514	.9337748
0.11	.9887779	.9775835	.9664167	.9552772	.9441652	.9330806
0.12	.9886519	.9773346	.9660480	.9547920	.9435666	.9323715
0.13	.9885229	.9770800	.9656712	.9542961	.9429549	.9316473
0.14	.9883910	.9768197	.9652858	.9537892	.9423299	.9309074
0.15	.9882561	.9765534	.9648918	.9532711	.9416909	.9301513
0.16	.9881179	.9762809	.9644887	.9527409	.9410377	.9293785
0.17	.9879764	.9760019	.9640762	.9521988	.9403697	.9285884
0.18	.9878316	.9757164	.9636541	.9516441	.9396864	.9277804
0.19	.9876832	.9754239	.9632218	.9510762	.9389872	.9269540
0.20	.9875312	.9751244	.9627792	.9504950	.9382716	.9261084

Table A.3 (Continued)

			θ			
P	0.01	0.02	0.03	0.04	0.05	0.06
0.21	.9873753	.9748174	.9623258	.9498998	.9375391	.9252429
0.22	.9872156	.9745028	.9618612	.9492901	.9367889	.9243571
0.23	.9870517	.9741802	.9613850	.9486652	.9360204	.9234499
0.24	.9868835	.9738494	.9608968	.9480249	.9352332	.9225206
0.25	.9867109	.9735099	.9603961	.9473684	.9344262	.9215686
0.26	.9865338	.9731616	.9598824	.9466951	.9335989	.9205929
0.27	.9863519	.9728039	.9593551	.9460042	.9327504	.9195926
0.28	.9861649	.9724366	.9588139	.9452954	.9318801	.9185668
0.29	.9859728	.9720592	.9582581	.9445676	.9309869	.9175144
0.30	.9857753	.9716714	.9576869	.9438202	.9300699	.9164345
0.31	.9855721	.9712726	.9571000	.9430524	.9291283	.9153260
0.32	.9853630	.9708625	.9564966	.9422632	.9281609	.9141876
0.33	.9851478	.9704404	.9558759	.9414519	.9271668	.9130183
0.34	.9849262	.9700061	.9552372	.9406176	.9261448	.9118166
0.35	.9846978	.9695586	.9545799	.9397590	.9250936	.9105812
0.36	.9844624	.9690977	.9539029	.9388752	.9240121	.9093108
0.37	.9842197	.9686226	.9532054	.9379652	.9228990	.9080037
0.38	.9839692	.9681326	.9524866	.9370277	.9217527	.9066584
0.39	.9837107	.9676271	.9517452	.9360613	.9205719	.9052731
0.40	.9834438	.9671052	.9509804	.9350649	.9193548	.9038461
0.41	.9831678	.9665664	.9501909	.9340369	.9180999	.9023755
0.42	.9828826	.9660096	.9493757	.9329758	.9168053	.9008592
0.43	.9825875	.9654338	.9485332	.9318801	.9154691	.8992951
0.44	.9822821	.9648382	.9476623	.9307479	.9140893	.8976808
0.45	.9819658	.9642218	.9467614	.9295774	.9126638	.8960139
0.46	.9816379	.9635834	.9458289	.9283668	.9111901	.8942918
0.47	.9812980	.9629218	.9448631	.9271136	.9096658	.8925117
0.48	.9809451	.9622357	.9438623	.9258161	.9080882	.8906706
0.49	.9805788	.9615236	.9428246	.9244713	.9064546	.8887652
0.50	.9801980	.9607844	.9417476	.9230769	.9047619	.8867925
0.51	.9798021	.9600159	.9406294	.9216301	.9030068	.8847482
0.52	.9793899	.9592169	.9394673	.9201278	.9011858	.8826291
0.53	.9789607	.9583854	.9382589	.9185668	.8992951	.8804305
0.54	.9785131	.9575191	.9370013	.9169436	.8973306	.8781478
0.55	.9780461	.9566161	.9356913	.9152542	.8952879	.8757764
0.56	.9775584	.9556738	.9343258	.9134948	.8931624	.8733108
0.57	.9770484	.9546896	.9329009	.9116608	.8909487	.8707454
0.58	.9765148	.9536608	.9314129	.9097473	.8886414	.8680739
0.59	.9759558	.9525841	.9298574	.9077491	.8862343	.8652896
0.60	.9753694	.9514563	.9282297	.9056604	.8837209	.8623853
0.61	.9747539	.9502734	.9265246	.9034749	.8810939	.8593530
0.62	.9741068	.9490316	.9247366	.9011858	.8783455	.8561841
0.63	.9734255	.9477261	.9228594	.8987855	.8754670	.8528691
0.64	.9727074	.9463519	.9208861	.8962656	.8724490	.8493976

Table A.3 (Continued)

			θ			
P	0.01	0.02	0.03	0.04	0.05	0.06
0.65	.9719495	.9449036	.9188092	.8936171	.8692810	.8457584
0.66	.9711483	.9433748	.9166203	.8908297	.8659517	.8419389
0.67	.9703000	.9417589	.9143102	.8878924	.8624484	.8379255
0.68	.9694003	.9400479	.9118684	.8847926	.8587570	.8337029
0.69	.9684444	.9382334	.9092833	.8815166	.8548621	.8292544
0.70	.9674267	.9363057	.9065421	.8780488	.8507462	.8245615
0.71	.9663413	.9342538	.9036299	.8743719	.8463901	.8196031
0.72	.9651811	.9320652	.9005305	.8704664	.8417721	.8143565
0.73	.9639380	.9297259	.8972251	.8663102	.8368679	.8087955
0.74	.9626029	.9272198	.8936924	.8618784	.8316498	.8028910
0.75	.9611651	.9245203	.8099002	.8571429	.8260870	.7966103
0.76	.9596122	.9216301	.8858448	.8520711	.8201439	.7899160
0.77	.9579301	.9185004	.8814699	.8466258	.8137803	.7827661
0.78	.9561018	.9151104	.8767461	.8407644	.8069498	.7751125
0.79	.9541074	.9114261	.8716303	.8344371	.7995993	.7668998
0.80	.9519231	.9074074	.8660714	.8275863	.7916667	.7580646
0.81	.9495204	.9030068	.8600093	.8201439	.7830803	.7485331
0.82	.9468650	.8981670	.8533724	.8120301	.7737557	.7382200
0.83	.9439147	.8928189	.8460749	.8031496	.7635934	.7270246
0.84	.9406176	.8868779	.8380130	.7933885	.7524753	.7148290
0.85	.9369085	.8802396	.8290598	.7826088	.7402598	.7014926
0.86	.9327052	.8727735	.8190591	.7706423	.7267760	.6868476
0.87	.9279019	.8643148	.8078155	.7572816	.7118156	.6706916
0.88	.9223602	.8546512	.7950820	.7422680	.6951220	.6527778
0.89	.9158958	.8435055	.7805414	.7252748	.6763755	.6328030
0.900	.9082569	.8305085	.7637796	.7058825	.6551725	.6103896
0.901	.9074161	.8290891	.7619615	.7037916	.6528984	.6079970
0.902	.9065596	.8276457	.7601152	.7016707	.6505941	.6055747
0.903	.9056871	.8261778	.7582401	.6995193	.6482590	.6031223
0.904	.9047982	.8246846	.7563355	.6973368	.6458926	.6006392
0.905	.9038924	.8231655	.7544005	.6951222	.6434940	.5981248
0.906	.9029692	.8126198	.7524346	.6928750	.6410628	.5955786
0.907	.9020281	.8200470	.7504370	.6905943	.6385980	.5929999
0.908	.9010686	.8184461	.7484068	.6882796	.6360993	.5903881
0.909	.9000901	.8168165	.7463434	.6859300	.6335658	.5877426
0.910	.8990920	.8151575	.7442458	.6835447	.6309967	.5850627
0.911	.8980736	.8134676	.7421130	.6811225	.6283909	.5823471
0.912	.8970346	.8117470	.7399445	.6786633	.6257485	.5795964
0.913	.8959742	.8099943	.7377393	.6761658	.6230682	.5768092
0.914	.8948918	.8082088	.7354965	.6736293	.6203493	.5739848
0.915	.8937866	.8063893	.7332149	.6710528	.6175909	.5711224
0.916	.8926579	.8045350	.7308936	.6684352	.6147921	.5682212
0.917	.8915049	.8026448	.7285315	.6657756	.6119521	.5652806
0.918	.8903269	.8007176	.7261276	.6630730	.6090698	.5622996

Table A.3 (Continued)

P	θ					
	0.01	0.02	0.03	0.04	0.05	0.06
0.919	.8891231	.7987525	.7236808	.6603264	.6061444	.5592776
0.920	.8878926	.7967483	.7211899	.6575346	.6031750	.5562133
0.921	.8866342	.7947034	.7186533	.6546961	.6001600	.5531059
0.922	.8853474	.7926172	.7160705	.6518106	.5970991	.5499551
0.923	.8840311	.7904882	.7134397	.6488765	.5939911	.5467594
0.924	.8826842	.7883151	.7107598	.6458925	.5908348	.5435181
0.925	.8813058	.7860963	.7080293	.6428573	.5876290	.5402301
0.926	.8798944	.7838307	.7052468	.6397696	.5843726	.5368943
0.927	.8784491	.7815165	.7024107	.6366281	.5810643	.5335098
0.928	.8769687	.7791521	.6995195	.6334314	.5777030	.5300755
0.929	.8754517	.7767361	.6965715	.6301779	.5742873	.5265903
0.930	.8738968	.7742666	.6935652	.6268661	.5708158	.5230528
0.931	.8723024	.7717417	.6904984	.6234940	.5672870	.5194618
0.932	.8706674	.7691599	.6873698	.6200609	.5636998	.5158168
0.933	.8689900	.7665189	.6841773	.6165645	.5600530	.5121159
0.934	.8672685	.7638168	.6809191	.6130033	.5563444	.5083581
0.935	.8655011	.7610516	.6775929	.6093753	.5525730	.5045420
0.936	.8636861	.7582207	.6741966	.6056785	.5487367	.5006661
0.937	.8618214	.7553220	.6707280	.6019111	.5448342	.4967291
0.938	.8599049	.7523530	.6671847	.5980712	.5408636	.4927295
0.939	.8579346	.7493110	.6635644	.5941563	.5368231	.4886659
0.940	.8559081	.7461933	.6598645	.5901645	.5327108	.4845366
0.941	.8538225	.7429967	.6560817	.5860928	.5285243	.4803396
0.942	.8516762	.7397190	.6522144	.5819399	.5242627	.4760742
0.943	.8494658	.7363566	.6482591	.5777029	.5199234	.4717382
0.944	.8471884	.7329063	.6442128	.5733791	.5155042	.4673298
0.945	.8448411	.7293643	.6400723	.5689658	.5110027	.4628473
0.946	.8424206	.7257271	.6358343	.5644603	.5064169	.4582886
0.947	.8399234	.7219909	.6314954	.5598596	.5017444	.4536519
0.948	.8373458	.7181515	.6270517	.5551606	.4969824	.4489351
0.949	.8346838	.7142046	.6224996	.5503603	.4921286	.4441363
0.950	.8319331	.7101456	.6178350	.5454552	.4871801	.4392530
0.951	.8290891	.7059690	.6130531	.5404413	.4821338	.4342826
0.952	.8261475	.7016708	.6081507	.5353162	.4769876	.4292239
0.953	.8231029	.6972452	.6031224	.5300755	.4717383	.4240740
0.954	.8199498	.6926862	.5979634	.5247152	.4663824	.4188303
0.955	.8166823	.6879880	.5926685	.5192312	.4609169	.4134902
0.956	.8132938	.6831437	.5872323	.5136192	.4553382	.4080510
0.957	.8097779	.6781467	.5816489	.5078746	.4496429	.4025101
0.958	.8061268	.6729895	.5759125	.5019928	.4438272	.3968644
0.959	.8023330	.6676644	.5700166	.4959685	.4378872	.3911110
0.960	.7983877	.6621630	.5639545	.4897968	.4318190	.3852467
0.961	.7942810	.6564753	.5577177	.4834709	.4256173	.3792674
0.962	.7900041	.6505940	.5513011	.4769874	.4192799	.3731717

Table A.3 (Continued)

			θ			
P	0.01	0.02	0.03	0.04	0.05	0.06
0.963	.7855458	.6445076	.5446958	.4703390	.4128009	.3669551
0.964	.7808940	.6382056	.5378929	.4635194	.4061759	.3606139
0.965	.7760360	.6316761	.5308838	.4565220	.3993996	.3541444
0.966	.7709576	.6249065	.5236586	.4493395	.3924669	.3475427
0.967	.7656436	.6178835	.5162076	.4419647	.3853722	.3408046
0.968	.7600772	.6105924	.5085196	.4343896	.3781099	.3339259
0.969	.7542398	.6030177	.5005833	.4266062	.3706740	.3269021
0.970	.7481114	.5951425	.4923866	.4186054	.3630580	.3197286
0.971	.7416688	.5869475	.4839153	.4103773	.3552545	.3123996
0.972	.7348887	.5784148	.4751575	.4019139	.3472584	.3049120
0.973	.7277431	.5695223	.4660973	.3932040	.3390616	.2972594
0.974	.7202016	.5602465	.4567188	.3842367	.3306562	.2894365
0.975	.7122305	.5505621	.4470050	.3750003	.3220342	.2814374
0.976	.7037920	.5404417	.4369374	.3654827	.3131873	.2732562
0.977	.6948435	.5298550	.4264966	.3556707	.3041063	.2648866
0.978	.6853375	.5187689	.4156611	.3455505	.2947821	.2563219
0.979	.6752201	.5071474	.4044084	.3351073	.2852046	.2475554
0.980	.6644306	.4949508	.3927137	.3243255	.2753633	.2385794
0.981	.6528983	.4821335	.3805492	.3131867	.2652461	.2293860
0.982	.6405465	.4686505	.3678889	.3016760	.2548436	.2199689
0.983	.6272831	.4544466	.3547002	.2897730	.2441423	.2103187
0.984	.6130036	.4394624	.3409495	.2774570	.2331292	.2004268
0.985	.5975862	.4236319	.3266000	.2647065	.2217904	.1902839
0.986	.5808895	.4068812	.3116118	.2514978	.2101113	.1798803
0.987	.5627473	.3891277	.2959411	.2378059	.1980763	.1692060
0.988	.5429633	.3702787	.2795403	.2236037	.1856688	.1582501
0.989	.5213043	.3502294	.2623573	.2088622	.1728714	.1470014
0.990	.4974902	.3288615	.2443345	.1935501	.1596653	.1354480
0.991	.4711794	.3060376	.2254067	.1776316	.1460291	.1235759
0.992	.4419648	.2816096	.2055088	.1610741	.1319447	.1113746
0.993	.4093336	.2553992	.1845617	.1438361	.1173879	.0988288
0.994	.3726491	.2272037	.1624800	.1258749	.1023346	.0859238
0.995	.3311061	.1967889	.1391692	.1071439	.0867589	.0726437
0.996	.2836681	.1638799	.1145221	.0875914	.0706321	.0589713
0.997	.2289912	.1281612	.0884235	.0671646	.0539266	.0448905
0.998	.1652778	.0892546	.0607399	.0458023	.0366095	.0303819
0.999	.0900857	.0467132	.0313221	.0234386	.0186466	.0154257

Table A.4   Bayesian posterior risk for the mother of an isolated male affected by an X-linked recessive disease. The mother also has a normal sons and b normal brothers. (The calculations assume that $\mu = \nu$ and that reproductive fitness, f, is zero).

Normal Sons	Normal Brothers					
	0	1	2	3	4	5
0	2/3	3/5	5/9	9/17	17/33	33/65
1	1/2	3/7	5/13	9/25	17/49	33/97
2	1/3	3/11	5/21	9/41	17/81	33/161
3	1/5	3/19	5/37	9/73	17/145	33/289
4	1/9	3/35	5/69	9/137	17/273	33/545
5	1/17	3/67	5/133	9/265	17/529	33/1057

Note: If the values under the $b = 0$ column are modified so that all of them have 2 as the numerator (2/3, 2/4, 2/6, 2/10, 2/18, 2/34), a progressive pattern becomes clear. The numerators can all be calculated using the formula $2^b + N/4$, and the denominators can all be calculated using the formula $2^b + 2^{a+b} + N/4$. The derivation of these formulae can be found in Table A.5.

Table A.5   Below is a general formula for the derivation of Bayesian posterior risks for X-linked recessive disorders (starting with the grandmother in case the mother has normal brothers). This formula also permits the calculation of risks when affected males can reproduce ($f > 0$ and $N > 4$, see Table 2.10), but does assume that the maternal grandfather of the affected male was normal.

Grandmother =	Carrier	Noncarrier
Prior probability	$N\mu$	1
Conditional probability		
b normal brothers	$\frac{1}{2}^b$	1
Joint probability	$\frac{1}{2}^b N\mu$	1

Mother =	Carrier	Noncarrier
Prior probability	$2\mu + \frac{1}{2}(\frac{1}{2}^b N\mu)$	1
	$= (2 + \frac{1}{2}^{b+1}N)\mu$	1
Conditional probability		
affected son	$\frac{1}{2}$	μ
a normal sons	$\frac{1}{2}^a$	1
Joint probability	$\frac{1}{2}^{a+1}(2 + \frac{1}{2}^{b+1}N)\mu$	μ
Posterior probability		

Carrier $= [\frac{1}{2}^{a+1}(2 + \frac{1}{2}^{b+1}N)]/(1 + [\frac{1}{2}^{a+1}(2 + \frac{1}{2}^{b+1}N)])$

Table A.5 (Continued)

This expression can be simplified to yield the formulae mentioned
in Table A.4 by the following steps:

Multiply top and bottom by 2^{a+1}

Carrier $= (2 + \frac{1}{2}^{b+1}N)/(2^{a+1} + 2 + \frac{1}{2}^{b+1}N)$

Multiply top and bottom by 2^{b+1}

Carrier $= (2^{b+2} + N)/(2^{a+b+2} + 2^{b+2} + N)$

Multiply top and bottom by $1/4$

Carrier $= (2^{b} + N/4)/(2^{a+b} + 2^{b} + N/4)$

N – coefficient of μ for female carrier risk (e.g., 4μ)

a = number of normal sons

b = number of normal brothers

The prior probabilities under the noncarrier column are technically equal to 1 minus the prior probabilities under the carrier column; however, since μ is very small, these are approximately equal to 1.

If the male and female mutation rates are known to be different, formula 2.6, $(2\mu + 2f\mu + 2\nu)/(1 - f)$, can be substituted for $N\mu$ under prior probability for the grandmother, and $\mu + \nu$ in place of the 2μ that allows for new mutations in the prior probability for the mother. Finally, if the maternal grandfather is not known to have been normal, the derivation could be modified in a manner similar to Table 2.12 using either $Y\mu$ (Table 2.13) or [(formula 2.6)/2] $+ \mu$ as the prior probability that an unknown grandfather would have been affected.

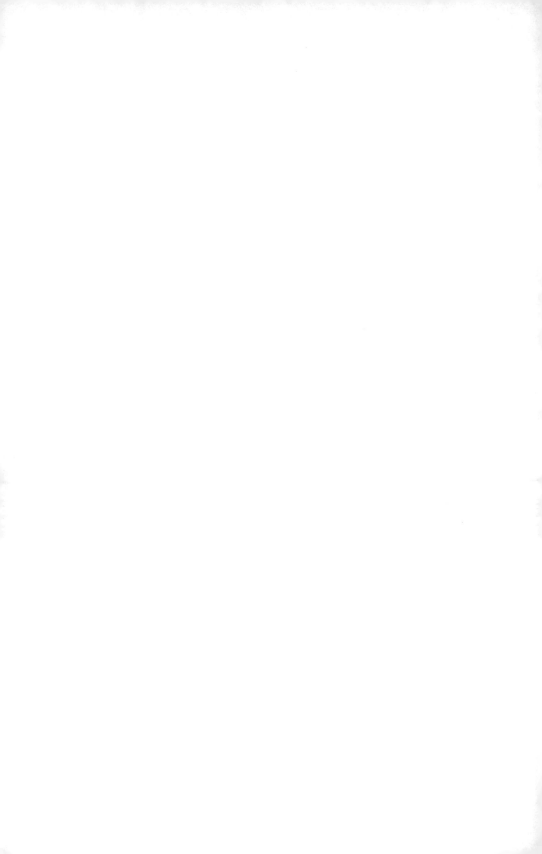

Glossary

It has been assumed throughout that most readers of this book would be very well versed in the terminology of human molecular genetics. However, for the benefit of any readers who are just starting to study this field, the following glossary is provided. Because it is written for a specific audience, the definitions are brief and not necessarily completely rigorous.

Alleles. Different forms of the same gene or locus, as in mutant and normal alleles of a gene, or A1 and A2 alleles at polymorphic locus A.

Allele-specific oligonucleotide (ASO). Short pieces of single-stranded DNA that are about 20 bases long. Under appropriate conditions, they will hybridize (stick) to only a perfectly complementary DNA sequence. The use of two ASOs that differ by a single base in the center of the sequence will permit discrimination between two alleles, since each ASO will hybridize to only one allele.

Autosomal. Pertaining to chromosomes other than X and Y (numbered chromosomes). Not involved in sex determination.

CA repeat (TG repeat). A polymorphism caused by a variable number of repeats of the dinucleotide sequence CA. Estimated to occur in 50,000 to 100,000 locations in the human genome. They are extremely useful tools for linkage studies because of their frequency, their high heterozygosity, and the fact that they are usually detected by PCR amplification.

Chimera/chimerism. The fusion of two embryos of dissimilar genotypes to form a hybrid containing two different cell lines (one not derived from the other as in mosaics).

cis. On the same side (i.e., on the same member of a pair of homologous chromosomes).

Compound heterozygote. A person who has two different mutant alleles, one on each of a pair of chromosomes. This person has no "normal" allele.

Disomy, uniparental. The inheritance of both copies of a chromosome pair from the same parent, instead of one copy from each parent. The most common mechanism is probably the correction of a trisomic cell line.

Dominant. Characters that are expressed in the heterozygous state (at the expense of a recessive trait).

Double mutation. Two independent mutations within the same allele or gene, either of which could cause disease.

DNA (deoxyribonucleic acid). The genetic material that contains coded information that can (*a*) be duplicated and (*b*) be decoded to form functional molecules within the cell.

Fitness, reproductive. A measure of the probability that an individual with a genetic disease will be able to reproduce. It is measured by counting the number of children born to affected people in comparison to their unaffected siblings.

Gene. A functional unit in a DNA sequence, which specifies the information necessary to perform a function (e.g., synthesize a specific protein).

Gene conversion. The products of meiosis in a Bb heterozygote would be expected to be 2 B gametes and 2 b gametes. Occasionally, meiosis results in 3 B and 1 b or 1 B and 3 b, giving the impression that one allele has been converted to the other. The mechanism is probably an excision and repair process that uses the wrong template to fill in the excised region. The result will be a DNA molecule that apparently contains a double crossover in a very small region.

Gene pool. The total collection of alleles in a population. This is normally used with reference to only one or a few loci at a time. If an island has 2 million inhabitants comprising 800 individuals affected by an autosomal recessive disease, 78,400 carriers, and 1,920,800 noncarriers, the gene pool of 4 million alleles contains $(800 * 2) + 78,400 = 80,000$ mutant alleles and $(1,920,800 * 2) + 78,400 = 3,920,000$ normal alleles.

Genetic lethal. A disease that prevents reproduction by an affected person and therefore causes the loss of that person's mutant alleles from the gene pool. The disease does not necessarily have to be fatal or diminish longevity to accomplish this.

Genome Project. See Human Genome Project.

Germline mosaicism/gonadal mosaicism. A person in whom a mitotic mutation occurred during embryogenesis will have two different cell lines (mosaic). If the gonads contain cells derived from both lines, the person will release gametes that contain the same haplotype with and without the mutation.

Haplotype. A collection of alleles on the same chromosome (in the *cis* configuration).

Hardy-Weinberg equilibrium. Under certain conditions (including no selection, random breeding, no migration into or out of the gene pool), the frequency of alleles in a gene pool will remain constant from one generation to the next. The frequencies of alleles are usually denoted p and q, and if applicable, p is used for the normal or dominant or more common allele and q for the mutant or recessive or less common allele. In a biallelic system, $p + q = 1.0$. Assuming random breeding, homozygotes would be expected to occur with frequencies of p^2 and q^2 and heterozygotes to occur with frequency $2pq$. For many rare recessive diseases, the frequency of the mutant allele q can be estimated by taking the square root of the frequency of affected individuals within the population. In the island population discussed above under gene pool, $q^2 = 800/2,000,000 = 0.0004$, so $q = 0.02$. If $q = 0.02$, $p = 0.98$, and from this we can calculate the expected number of carriers and noncarriers on the island (carriers $= 2 * p * q *$ population $= 2 * 0.98 * 0.02 * 2,000,000 = 78,400$; noncarriers $= p^2 *$ population $= 0.98 * 0.98 * 2,000,000 = 1,920,800$).

Hemizygous. Pertaining to genes on the single X chromosome in males. Since males have only one X chromosome, they cannot be homozygous or heterozygous.

Heteroplasmic. A cell that contains mitochondria with two or more different forms of mitochondrial DNA.

Heterozygosity. The expected frequency with which random individuals will be heterozygous at a particular locus.

Heterozygous. Possessing two different alleles at a given locus.

Homoplasmic. A cell that contains mitochondria of only one genotype.

Homozygous. Possessing two copies of the same allele at a given locus.

Human Genome Project. A multinational project to obtain first a fine-resolution genetic map of all human chromosomes and an ordered array of cloned fragments that encompass the entire genome followed by the complete DNA sequence of all of the chromosomes. At its beginning in 1990, it was envisaged that this would require 15 years to complete. This can be broken down (very crudely) into efforts in mapping, cloning, and sequencing. In the first 5 years, a comprehensive genetic map would be constructed with an average space between markers of 2 cM. During the second 5 years, this map would be refined to a 1 cM map or better. During the first 5 years, cloning and physical mapping would start to give complete coverage of the human genome with overlapping, ordered cloned fragments; during the second 5 years, this task would be completed. During the first 5 years, 1% of the total genome would be sequenced; during the second 5 years, 10% of the genome would be sequenced; during the last 5 years, all of the remainder would be sequenced. This primary DNA sequence will be an invaluable sourcebook for all aspects of the health sciences. Perhaps it should be emphasized that it will take much longer to truly understand the sequence than it will take to obtain it.

Imprinting. A temporary means of marking or modifying a DNA sequence such that its expression is different from an unimprinted or differently imprinted allele. Methylation of bases is probably the most frequent mechanism of imprinting. Imprinting is stable during mitosis (i.e., also applied to nascent DNA molecules during cell division), but is removed prior to or during meiosis (but could be reapplied or reversed).

Linkage. When alleles at two loci are coinherited at a frequency greater than that expected under independent assortment, the loci are said to be linked. The loci must be on the same chromosome to be linked.

Linkage disequilibrium. A nonrandom association of specific alleles of linked genes in the gametes of a population.

Location score. A measure of the probability that a test locus resides at a specified position within a series of previously mapped loci. The result of multipoint linkage analysis.

Locus. A specified position on a chromosome. A locus may be a gene, but does not have to be. Often used to refer simultaneously to the corresponding positions on a pair of homologous chromosomes.

Lod score. The abbreviation for logarithm of the odds. A measure of the odds ratio obtained by dividing the likelihood that two loci are linked at a specific recombination fraction by the likelihood that they are unlinked.

Mendelian. Following an inheritance pattern predicted by Mendel's laws.

Mendel's laws (paraphrased). (1) The law of segregation. The two alleles at any locus remain discrete and are separated at meiosis, so only one allele is placed into each gamete. (2) The law of independent assortment. Members of different pairs of alleles are assorted independently during gamete formation (provided that they are unlinked; linkage was not known at the time that Mendel formulated this law).

Microsatellite. Regions that are repeated many times throughout the genome that contain a very simple repetitive motif. *See* CA repeat.

Mosaic. Containing two different cell lines, one of which is derived from the other (or both are derived from a common progenitor).

Mu (μ). The symbol used to represent the mutation rate in females. When the mutation rates are known to be equal, or when differences in mutation rates between the sexes are ignored, μ may be used to designate the mutation rate in both sexes.

Mutation. Any change in the sequence of a DNA molecule. A mutation may result in disease if it occurs in the small fraction of the genome that contains coding sequences, or it may be a totally harmless polymorphism. Mutation forms the basis for the difference between alleles. Some mutations are even beneficial and may be the substrate for positive natural selection.

Nu ν. The symbol used to designate the mutation rate in males.

Null allele. An invisible allele usually caused by the deletion of a polymorphic site. An individual with a null allele is functionally hemizygous for that locus and may be mistyped as being homozygous for the visible allele.

Penetrance. The proportion of individuals with a specified genotype who show the expected phenotype (under apparently identical conditions). Usually used in the sense of nonpenetrance to describe asymptomatic heterozygotes for an autosomal dominant disease.

PFGE (pulsed field gel electrophoresis). A method of gel electrophoresis used to separate very large DNA molecules. Its success depends upon periodically changing the direction of the applied electric field (pulsed field), so that the DNA molecules periodically have to change the direction in which they are migrating through the gel.

Phase (known/unknown). A person is phase-known when a study of the parents has shown that there is only one possible arrangement of his or her alleles into specific haplotypes at the loci of interest (i.e., we know unambiguously which alleles are in the *cis* arrangement on the same chromosome). A person is phase-unknown (but phase may be inferred) when we have been unable to prove the arrangement of his or her alleles into haplotypes by a study of the parents.

PIC (polymorphism information content). A measure of the probability that a locus will be informative in linkage analysis. To be informative, the individual must be heterozygous, and the spouse and children must have genotypes that allow the determination of the source of each allele (e.g., if both parents and the child are heterozygous A1/A2, the mating is uninformative because we do not know which parent contributed which allele in the child).

Poly(A) mutations. At the end of many genes there is a signal indicating that a chain of adenine (A) residues should be added to the end of the mRNA. This chain is frequently about 200 A residues long on a nascent mRNA molecule, and it is thought that every time a ribosome reads the mRNA during protein synthesis it removes a few As from the end, thus shortening the chain. When the chain gets too short, the mRNA is degraded. In this way, the life span of an mRNA molecule can be controlled. If a person has a mutation in the poly(A) signal, the poly(A) tail will not be added to the mRNA. Although the mRNA specifies a normal protein product, it is very unstable, and protein deficiency may result.

Polymorphism. Occurring in different forms. Usually applied to harmless variants rather than to disease-causing mutations.

Positional cloning. A process whereby the locus for a genetic disease has been demonstrated to be confined within a small region of a chromosome by analysis of closely linked flanking markers. These markers define a candidate region (frequently 1 to 10 million base pairs of DNA). Searching for expressed genes throughout the candidate region will yield cDNA molecules. Analysis of each cDNA for features expected for the gene of interest will usually identify a candidate cDNA. The cDNA will then be sequenced, the intron/exon boundaries determined, and (eventually) the genomic DNA cloned and sequenced. To prove that the cDNA comes from a locus that is involved in a genetic disease usually also requires finding mutations in affected individuals that can explain the cause of the disease as well as studies in cell cultures to show that the normal cDNA can correct the deficiency in mutant cells (recessive diseases) or that the mutant cDNA can cause problems in normal cells (dominant diseases).

Private variant. A rare mutation or polymorphism. May be unique to one family.

Recessive. A character that is expressed only in the homozygous state. A character that is not expressed in the presence of a dominant trait.

Restriction enzyme. A bacterial enzyme that cuts DNA when a specific sequence of bases is present. These sequences, called restriction sites, are usually between 4 and 8 bases long. A mutation that falls within this sequence will alter the pattern of cleavage by that restriction enzyme and generate an RFLP.

Reverse genetics. A process whereby random DNA sequence is screened for features associated wtih genes. If such features are identified, analysis of the DNA sequence will predict protein sequence and (eventually) protein function. In this process, the phenotype would be predicted purely from the DNA sequence. It is expected that this process will become routine in the late stages of the Human Genome Project or following its completion, when we start to understand what the sequence means.

RFLP (restriction fragment length polymorphism). Variation in the length of DNA fragments from a given locus following treatment with a restriction enzyme. The variation in length may be caused by the creation of a new restriction site, by abolition of an existing one, or by insertions or deletions that vary the length of DNA between constant enzyme sites (see VNTR).

Syntenic. On the same DNA strand. All linked loci are necessarily syntenic.

Theta (θ) and $\hat{\theta}$. The symbol used to denote the recombination fraction, when it is known, is θ. The symbol used to denote the best estimate of θ based upon current evidence during linkage studies is $\hat{\theta}$. The best estimate will be the value of θ at which the lod score has its highest value.

trans. On the opposite side (i.e., on different members of a pair of homologous chromosomes).

VNTR (variable number of tandem repeats). A type of polymorphism caused by the presence of a variable number of repetitive units between two restriction sites. Because the mutation does not affect the sequence of the restriction sites, it is usually possible to detect VNTR polymorphisms with several different restriction enzymes. The repeat unit is larger than in CA repeats and other microsatellites.

X-linked. On the X chromosome and therefore following a distinctive pattern of inheritance.

Z *and* $\hat{Z}$. The symbols used to denote the lod score and the maximum lod score, respectively.

References

Bakker, E., Veenema, H., den Dunnen, J. T., van Broeckhoven, C., Grootscholten, P. M., Bonten, E. J., van Ommem, G. J. B., and Pearson, P. L. 1989. Germinal mosaicism increases the recurrence risk for "new" Duchenne muscular dystrophy mutations. *J. Med. Genet.* 26:553–559.

Beaudet, A. L., Feldman, G. L., Fernbach, S. D., Buffone, G. J., and O'Brien, W. E. 1989. Linkage disequilibrium, cystic fibrosis, and genetic counseling. *Am. J. Hum. Genet.* 44:319–326.

Bridge, P. J., and Lillicrap, D. P. 1989. Molecular diagnosis of the fragile X [Fra(X)] syndrome: Calculation of risks based on flanking DNA markers in small phase-unknown families. *Am. J. Med. Genet.* 33:92–99.

Bundey, S. 1978. Calculation of genetic risks in Duchenne muscular dystrophy by geneticists in the United Kingdom. *J. Med. Genet.* 15:249–253.

Childs, B., Holtzman, N. A., Kazazian, H. H. Jr., and Valle, D. L., eds. 1988. *Molecular Genetics in Medicine.* New York: Elsevier.

Conneally, P. M., Edwards, J. H., Kidd, K. K., Lalouel, J.-M., Morton, N. E., Ott, J., and White, R. 1985. Report of the Committee on Methods of Linkage Analysis and Reporting. Eighth International Workshop on Human Gene Mapping. *Cytogenet. Cell Genet.* 40:356–359.

Connor, J. M., and Ferguson-Smith, M. A. 1987. *Essential Medical Genetics.* 2d ed. Oxford: Blackwell Scientific Publications.

Côté, G. B. 1989a. The cis-trans effects of crossing-over on the penetrance and expressivity of dominantly inherited disorders. *Ann. Génét.* 32:132–135.

Côté, G. B. 1989b. Wilm's tumour and related syndromes: A unifying theory. *Ann. Génét.* 32:69–72.

Côté, G. B., and Gyftodimou, J. 1991. Twinning and mitotic crossing-over: Some possibilities and their implications. *Am. J. Hum. Genet.* 49:120–130.

Edwards, J. H. 1976. The interpretation of lod scores in linkage analysis. *Cytogenet. Cell Genet.* (HGM3) 16:289–293.

Estivill, X., Farrall, M., Williamson, R., Ferrari, M., Seia, M., Giunta, A. M., Novelli, G., Potenza, L., Dallapicolla, B., Borgo, G., Gasparini, P., Pignatti, P. F., De Benedetti, L., Vitale, E., Devoto, M., and Romeo, G. 1988. Linkage disequilibrium between cystic fibrosis and linked DNA polymorphisms in Italian families: A collaborative study. *Am. J. Hum. Genet.* 43:23–28.

Friedman, J. M. 1985. Genetic counseling for autosomal dominant diseases with a negative family history. *Clin. Genet.* 27:68–71.

Graham, G. E., MacLeod, P. M., Lillicrap, D. P., and Bridge, P. J. 1992. Gonadal mosaicism in a family with adrenoleukodystrophy: Molecular diagnosis of carrier status among daughters of a gonadal mosaic when direct detection of the mutation is not possible. *J. Inherited Metab. Dis.* 15:68–74.

Grimm, T. 1984. Genetic counseling in Becker type X-linked muscular dystrophy. I. Theoretical considerations. *Am. J. Med. Genet.* 18:713–718.

Hall, J. G. 1990. Genomic imprinting: Review and relevance to human diseases. *Am. J. Hum. Genet.* 46:857–873.

Kadasi, L. 1989. Estimating the error rate in DNA diagnosis with linked markers. *Hum. Hered.* 39:67–74.

Kazazian, H. H., Jr., and Antonarakis, S. E. 1988. The varieties of mutation. In: Childs, B., Holtzman, N. A., Kazazian, H. H., Jr., and Valle, D. L., eds. *Molecular Genetics in Medicine.* New York: Elsevier, pp. 43–67.

Koeberl, D. D., Bottema, C. D. K., Ketterling, R. P., Bridge, P. J., Lillicrap, D. P., and Sommer, S. S. 1990. Mutations causing hemophilia B: Direct estimate of the underlying rates of spontaneous germ-line transitions, transversions, and deletions in a human gene. *Am. J. Hum. Genet.* 47:202–217.

Lander, E. S., Green, P., Abrahamson, J., Barlow, A., Daly, M. J., Lincoln, S. E., and Newburg, L. 1987. MAPMAKER: an interactive computer package for constructing primary genetic linkage maps of experimental and natural populations. *Genomics* 1:174–181.

Lathrop, G. M., and Lalouel, J. M. 1984. Easy calculations of lod scores and genetic risks on small computers. *Am. J. Hum. Genet.* 36:460–465.

Maynard-Smith, S., Penrose, L. S., and Smith, C. A. B. 1961. *Mathe-*

matical Tables for Research Workers in Human Genetics. London: J & A Churchill.

Milunsky, A. 1992. *Heredity and Your Family's Health.* Baltimore: Johns Hopkins University Press.

Murphy, E. A., and Chase, G. A. 1975. *Principles of Genetic Counselling.* Chicago: Year Book Medical Publishers.

Ott, J. 1974. Estimation of the recombination fraction in human pedigrees: Efficient computation of the likelihood for human linkage studies. *Am. J. Hum. Genet.* 26:588–597.

Ott, J. 1985. *Analysis of Human Genetic Linkage.* Baltimore: Johns Hopkins University Press.

Ott, J. 1991. *Analysis of Human Genetic Linkage.* Rev. ed. Baltimore: Johns Hopkins University Press.

Passos-Bueno, M. R., Bakker, E., Kneppers, A. L. J., Takata, R. I., Rapaport, D., den Dunnen, J. T., Zatz, M., and van Ommen, G. J. B. 1992. Different mosaicism frequencies for proximal and distal Duchenne muscular dystrophy (DMD) mutations indicate different etiology and recurrence risk. *Am. J. Hum. Genet.* 51:1150–1155.

Round, A. P. 1989. SCHESIS: Computation in a multipoint linkage analysis program. In: Elston, R. C., et al., eds. *Multipoint Mapping and Linkage Based upon Affected Pedigree Members.* Genetic Analysis Workshop 6. New York: Alan R. Liss, pp. 69–74.

Round, A. P. 1992. A novel pedigree plotting algorithm. *Cytogenet. Cell Genet.* 59:133–135.

Roychoudhury, A. K., and Nei, M. 1988. *Human Polymorphic Genes: Worldwide Distribution.* Oxford: Oxford University Press.

Sherman, S. L., Takaesu, N., Freeman, S. B., Grantham, M., Phillips, C., Blackston, R. D., Jacobs, P. A., Cockwell, A. E., Freeman, V., Uchida, I., Mikkelsen, M., Kurnit, D. M., Buraczynska, M., Keats, B. J. B., and Hassold, T. J. 1991. Trisomy 21: Association between reduced recombination and nondisjunction. *Am. J. Hum. Genet.* 49:608–620.

White, M. B., Leppert, M., Nielsen, D., Zielenski, L., Gerrard, B., Stewart, C., and Dean, M. 1991. A de novo cystic fibrosis mutation: CGA (Arg) to TGA (Stop) at codon 851 of the CFTR gene. *Genomics* 11:778–779.

Wijsman, E. M. 1991. Recurrence risk of a new dominant mutation in children of unaffected parents. *Am. J. Hum. Genet.* 48:654–661.

Young, I. D. 1991. *Introduction to Risk Calculation in Genetic Counselling.* New York: Oxford University Press.

Index

About the Author

Peter J. Bridge was born in Newton-le-Willows, England. He obtained a B.Sc. (Honours in Biochemistry) from the University of Manchester Institute of Science and Technology in 1978 and a Ph.D. in Biochemistry from the University of Regina, in Regina, Canada, in 1985. After a postdoctoral fellowship studying plant genetics, he moved to Queen's University to begin studying human molecular genetics.

Bridge has served as assistant professor and associate professor in the Departments of Pathology, Paediatrics, and Biology at Queen's University, and as co-director of the DNA Diagnostic Laboratory at Kingston General Hospital, in Kingston, Ontario. He is currently associate professor in the Departments of Pediatrics and Pathology at Memorial University, St. John's, Newfoundland.

Bridge is a Fellow of the Canadian College of Medical Geneticists (CCMG). He has chaired the molecular genetics committee of the CCMG since 1991 and has served as the chief examiner in molecular genetics for the examinations committee. In 1992 he was admitted as a Founding Fellow of the new American College of Medical Genetics.

Library of Congress Cataloging-in-Publication Data

Bridge, Peter J., 1957–
     The calculation of genetic risks : worked examples in DNA
diagnostics / Peter J. Bridge.
          p.   cm.
     Includes bibliographical references and index.
     ISBN 0-8018-4678-1 (hc : alk. paper)
     1. Genetic disorders—Diagnosis. 2. Genetic disorders—Risk
factors. 3. Health risk assessment. 4. Risk Factors. I. Title.
     [DNLM: 1. Hereditary Diseases—epidemiology. 2. Hereditary
Diseases—genetics. 3. DNA Probes—diagnostic use. 4. Molecular
Probe Techniques.   QZ 50 B851c 1994]
RB155.6.B75   1994
616'.042—dc20
DNLM/DLC
for Library of Congress   93-25080